MW01230495

The Journey Into Consciousness

The Journey Into Consciousness

A Guide to Reach Your Highest Potential

Eric Banter, C-IAYT
Amy Banter, MD

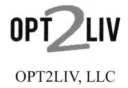

OPT2LIV, LLC

Published by OPT2LIV, LLC, Fishers, Indiana

Design and Production by Jacob Banter, Banter Productions, LLC.

Photography is by Jacob Banter.

OPT2LIV also publishes its books in a variety of electronic formats. For more information about OPT2LIV products, please visit our web site at www.opt2liv.com

Library of Congress Cataloging-in-Publication Data:

The Journey into Consciousness: a guide to reach your highest potential / Eric Banter / Amy Banter

ISBN-13 978-1-965000-00-7 (ebook)
ISBN-13 978-1-965000-01-4 (paperback)
ISBN-13-978-1-965000-02-1(hardback)

This book is dedicated to those ready
to raise the consciousness for all of humanity

Table of Contents

Acknowledgments

We would like to thank our kids, Lucas, Jacob, and Lucy for being in our lives and for lifting up our road of loving consciousness. It is through a richness of life experiences with you that our Journey into Consciousness has evolved. We would like to thank their significant others Elaine, Clair, and Matt respectively for being in our live's as loving Soulmates to our kids. Your relationships are a witness to the power of kindness, respect and love, and an example for those around you. To our parents for raising us with such love that our inner spark of consciousness was so easily lit at a young age. To our family and friends that have shown us the depths of true communion with one another that always lead us into laughter, joy, and love. To our Catholic Faith that has been our foundation of spiritual growth. To our friends in Cursillo that are a spark for the Holy Spirit and a willingness to share their spark with others. To the collection of clergy and laity that have a quest for Communion with all people. To our yoga teachers for sharing their knowledge and experiences of the art-of-yoga with us that has enhanced our awareness of the integration of the Soul into the body. To our yoga students that have kept an open heart and mind to our teachings, allowing them to experience an accelerated rate of their own spiritual evolution. To our patients that believe in us to give them their highest quality of life possible. To all pioneers in medicine that continue to lift up the care of patients and the efficacy of medicine through researching the complexities of the body and then developing and applying techniques and modalities of care that are bringing patients into homeostasis (balance), so that they can realize their highest quality of life possible.

Preface

Our Souls found each other in 1983 at the ages of 14 and 16. The moment we met there was a deep Knowing that we were meant to be together on this life journey. At the time we married in our early 20's, Eric worked as a mechanical engineer and Amy started medical school. Navigating life through marriage, the corporate world, the traditional medical system, raising 3 children, juggling full-time demanding careers, and navigating the loss of loved ones along the way has led us on our own Journey into Consciousness and the evolution of this book.

We were both blessed to be born into very faith filled Catholic families as well as to discover yoga at a young age. We strove to integrate this spiritual foundation into our own family. We raised our children in Catholic schools and were very integrated in our church and mission trips.

We became caught up in the typical quest to live the so-called "American Dream". By our 30's Amy was a full-time family physician and co-director of a family medicine residency program and Eric had started his own thriving business. We had achieved the "American Dream" – 3 beautiful children, a large home, expensive cars, a nanny, a housekeeper, all the material things we wanted, lots of wonderful friends, very successful careers, lavish vacations, big parties, and yet we were reaching a point of desperation. That's right, DESPERATION!

That may sound extreme, but our pace of life had gotten so crazy we could barely breathe. Don't get us wrong, we had a "good life", actually a "great life". But somehow we had gotten too overloaded. We lost the margins in our life and soon we realized there were more days of feeling stressed, tired, and overwhelmed than present and in the moment. We both felt an "Inner Knowing" that there was more that we were to be doing. But how could we add more? We were striving to meet society's expectations, succumbing to the pressures of this American culture by trying to BE the "American Dream", while in reality it was steering us further and further away from our true purpose here on Earth and God's dream for our journey together.

Our transition began after Eric's Dad became sick, very sick with terminal prostate cancer. Suddenly we both had an Awakening of the precious gift of life. We began to slow down enough to hear that voice in our heads which over time we realized was actually God guiding us down the path we were truly meant to follow, one of love and service to our family and those around us. So we quit our jobs, sold most of our belongings, cut our income in half and moved to be closer to family and to start up a wellness center focusing on helping others "break the pace" and find balance, joy and health in their lives.

This leap of faith seemed a bit crazy to those around us. They would ask, "Why would you want to step away from this wonderful life and leave all of your wonderful stuff?". This included leaving our high salary jobs and big home to go to a tiny 2 bedroom home, living paycheck to paycheck, moving the kids, reduced spending, and completely changing our lifestyle. During this time there was anxiety and even questioning if we did the right thing, but deep down we know that these changes were part of a new chapter in our life and would lead us even closer to our purpose.

Amy started her own private practice giving her the autonomy to practice medicine the way she wanted. Eric received his yoga therapy certification in 2006. We opened a yoga and wellness studio and soon after a yoga school with his Mom, Linda. Eric advanced his training and became one of only a few 1,000 hour certified Yoga Therapists in the country. Amy and all 3 of our kids eventually become certified yoga instructors and have continued to weave their spirituality and yoga into their lives and careers.

It was during this new chapter in our life that we realized how important it is to settle our minds, take time out to slow our life, and truly schedule more quiet time. That's right, it has to be scheduled! Living in this modern society can be such a distraction and striving to live a conscious life is very countercultural. We see it today with our patients as they too struggle to be on a health journey with us while trying to keep up with society, kids schedules and work expectations.

As we reflect back on these years, slowing down and being able to actually "be in the moment" with our children, our families, our friends and our patients has been the greatest gift not only to us but hopefully to future generations as these experiences perpetuate this into others lives.

As part of Eric's daily meditation routine, he began writing "muses" or journal entries capturing what came to his consciousness during his meditation practice. We definitely don't claim to have all the answers for this Journey into Consciousness perfected, but we have spent the past 20 years educating ourselves and integrating changes that we believe will help you along your journey.

It is our hope that this guidebook and these 108 muses can help inspire you and offer clarity on your own personal Journey into Consciousness.

Introduction

This book is written to encourage and support individuals along their Journey into Consciousness, where *Consciousness* is our ability to hold a state of harmony between our body, mind, and Soul.

The human form has been in a dance with Consciousness for ten to twenty thousand years, when our lens of duality, that which keeps us separated from God, started to become more transparent, allowing us to realize the collection of all the things God has created as infinitely interconnected. This non-dual state of mind is what allows us to begin to parse out aspects of the Infinite with our finite mind, to imagine a Creator that is working with us at all times to help us see clearly with our mind[1] how our actions can perfectly align with the evolution[2] of Her Creation.[3]

This book is written inclusively for all people across all beliefs and religions. It is not designed to cause someone to change their beliefs or religion, but merely to enhance and accelerate their current Journey into Consciousness, moving us from passive into active participation. *Active*

---

[1] It is the mind that has to be refined and awakened; Christians call this Christ Consciousness. Hindus see that the mind needs to be destroyed and reborn, Shiva.

[2] There is a force at work in the Universe that is constantly focused on creating newness, improving, evolving, and this form is called many things, including but not limited to the Holy Spirit, Prana, Chi, or Vishnu.

[3] The feminine sense of God is used in the book for it more easily aligns with the feminine characteristics of care, compassion, and love

participation means that we are willing to do our part to bring the body, mind, and Soul into One!

This book is separated into two parts. The first part is a guide to help us evolve spiritually, through showing us how to refine, surrender, and remove dis-ease from the body and mind, so that the Soul, or God Consciousness, can be more prevalent in our life, and the second part is a culmination of Conscious Thoughts to help us focus and attune the mind for the day.

Consciousness is directly tied to our health. As healthcare providers since 1991, we have witnessed time and again that our state of health can only become optimal when we connect the physical, mental, and emotional states of our being. In our medical practice, we focus on what creates health versus just diagnosing and treating disease (dis-ease). We focus on the 4 Pillars of Health: Breathe~Eat~Move~Sleep. Studies show that 80 percent of disease can be prevented through our lifestyle and addressing these 4 Pillars.[4] There is so much solid evidence on this, yet most of us have difficulty putting it into practice. Optimizing these 4 Pillars of Health is necessary as we begin to refine, surrender, and remove dis-ease from the body and mind. We must be intentional and make conscious decisions in life every day. This is the reason we were called to write this book. We have come across so many patients and clients who are on this journey of discovery. And by choosing this book, you

---

[4] Willett W. C. Balancing Lifestyle and Genomics Research for Disease Prevention. Science. 2002;296:695–98.

have proven that you, too, are walking a Journey into Consciousness.

We have laid out the guide that follows to help you personally tap into an awareness of the Infinite, refine your Finite, and form your own Infinite Being. And finally, it is our hope that through this book, we will help guide your personal journey toward a life filled with Consciousness, Health, Peace, Joy, and Love!

Part I: Guide to Spiritual Evolution

Chapter 1: Called into the Infinite

Hearing the Whisper

We are designed as Infinite beings and therefore are all called to participate in the Infinite, in God's Creation. If we choose to follow this calling, we will be participating at the highest level of our existence, where our Infinite Soul and physical purpose meet. This journey is the "Road Less Traveled," because to stay on this path, we have to learn to surrender our powerful instincts of fear and survival. This is essential, for it is through our deepest surrender that our Soul can be seen in the mind, allowing us to witness the Collective Consciousness of God's Creation. It is from this awakening, this Knowing, or this Divine Discontent, and the Grace of God that we take our first step toward renewal. From this day forward, we will be forever initiated into the journey toward Consciousness, where our actions align with the Creator and we play a part in "Positively Impacting the Face of the Earth."

What is the origin of our whisper? The finite world would say it comes from the brain and hence the mind, but science is helping us to see through a new lens. New findings in the field of quantum physics, the study of energy and matter dating back to the 1800s, are showing us that there is much more to our universe than we can sense, measure, or even imagine. It has been proven that as of today, 4 percent of the energy in the Universe is seen and measurable, and 96 percent of the energy is unseen and unmeasurable.[5] Therefore, 4 percent of the whisper comes from our finite mind, the seen realm, and 96 percent comes from the Unseen realm. We all have an inner Knowing of this Unseen realm from our evolving sense of intuition, giving us a peek into the Collective Consciousness of God's Creation.

Since Consciousness is evolving at an ever increasing rate[6], it will be our responsibility to recognize our journey within this growth. Some are already open to its whisper inside their heart and mind, while others find it to be confusing and scary. This disoriented state can present as a behavioral health condition, such as anxiety or depression, which is increasing amongst millennials at an alarming rate. A 2018 Blue Cross Blue Shield report highlighted that major depression diagnoses for millennials had risen 47 percent in 2013[7] compared to a comprehensive rate of 4 percent for all behavioral therapies.[8]

This evolved mind will have to take on characteristics of a new world explorer like Christopher Columbus, Marco Polo, or Sacagawea. This exploring mind will need to seek out new knowledge, go into unknown territories, document what it finds, and then share its findings with

[5] What's 96 Percent of the Universe Made Of?, www.space.com, May 12, 2011.
[6] Richard Rohr, *New Great Themes of Scripture*, 2010.
[7] Christopher Curley, "Why Millennial Depression Is on the Rise," Healthline, March 12, 2019.
[8] IBISWorld, "Behavioral Therapists in the US Market Size 2002-2025."

others, so that their Journey into Consciousness will be less treacherous, scary, and unknown.

The journey to find the whisper begins by finding stillness. "Be Still and Know God."[9] This is not a statement; this is a fact! When we are still, and we start to get good at it, the subtleties of our Soul's whisper are realized, lighting our path for the day. This is the easiest way to find God's purpose for us, and when we do, we are rewarded with pure joy.

What is the next stage in the evolution of human beings? Life on Earth began about 3.8 billion years ago, and about 200 million years ago, early mammals developed.[10] Our most recent advancement began around 10–20 thousand years ago when our brain's powerful survival instincts softened to uncover our next state of being, Consciousness. This faculty gives us an opportunity to be conscious of what it means to love another. Of course, we have all experienced the love of our family and friends, but God calls us into a deeper love, a love for all beings.

> Love one another as I have loved you.
> —John 15:12, Christian[11]

---

[9] Psalm 46:10

[10] Michael Marshall, "New Timeline: The Evolution of Life," newscientist.com, July 14, 2009

[11] "Love is a gift of one's inner most Soul to another so both can be whole" (Buddha)
"Love your neighbor as yourself—I am God" (Leviticus 19:18, Judaism)
"This is the sum of duty; do naught onto others what you would not have them do unto you" (Mahabharata 5, 1517, Hindu)

This type of love is all-inclusive compared to the specific and special love we have for our family. When we are able to hold this comprehensive state of love for another for longer than a few seconds, we accelerate the rate of our evolution. In this state, we are operating on a different vibration, and some would call it Agape,[12] our natural state of love for another being. This state holds the key to being in pure communion with God, because when we are in communion with another, we share the pieces of Consciousness that we have uncovered with the other, doubling or tripling our own Consciousness. When the day comes that we are all in communion with one another, we will be one step closer to realizing our Eternal God and the Infinite Universe.

Life as we know it was not designed to be personal. It was designed to be communal. When we make it personal, we narrow our full potential in life. To live an individual life is to live a self-serving life, one that works to satisfy our desires and wants, whereas a communal life is one of connectedness and service. I often think of Mother Teresa's example of service before self.

> Spread love everywhere you go. Let no one ever
> come to you without leaving happier.
> —Mother Teresa

"Serve Allah, and join not any partners with Him; and do good- to parents, kinsfolk, orphans, those in need, neighbors who are near, neighbors who are strangers, and companion by your side, the wayfarer (ye meet)" (Qur'an 4:36, Islam)

[12] "Agape," Wikipedia, https://en.wikipedia.org/wiki/Agape

Mother Teresa founded the Missionaries of Charity, in which, as of 2023, over 5,750 nuns served in 139 countries in 760 homes, with 244 of these homes in India, to help people dying of HIV/AIDS, leprosy, and tuberculosis. Their vows include chastity, poverty, obedience, and to give wholehearted free service to the poorest of the poor.[13]

This is just the opposite of how many in advanced societies live today, where our freedom has given way to gluttony, pride, and personal satisfaction. When we lose the connection with God's whisper inside, it is easy to fall into a mind of survival. This is also part of God's design, but we are called to be much more—we are called to be the Mother Teresas of today. We are called to move beyond our personal desires and wants and to believe in the communal journey that is ready to be discovered and created, our Consciousness.

This book is designed to help you refine your mind, find your whisper, and prepare for a journey of newness, clarity, and bliss. Thanks for daring to be a New World Explorer!

The Complexities of Our Body

The path toward Consciousness should begin each day with us marveling at the fact that we are one of the most

---

[13] Missionaries of Charity, Wikipedia, en.wikipedia.org/wiki/Missionaries_of_Charity

complex living things on this planet and that our potential is limitless, because our life is being sustained from an Infinite source, our Soul. The more conscious we are of this Infinite potential, the greater our desire to work toward this positive change in our life. In this state, we realize the need to align our finite, the little self, with our Infinite, the big Self.

Looking outward, it is truly a miracle that we are alive on this earth in the universe at this time, that we have an atmosphere protecting us from harmful sun radiation, and the perfect balance of air, water, and food to sustain us. Looking inward, science tells us that we are very complex and that there is still much to learn. If we just look at the chemistry of the body, there are about 3.0×10^{13} cells[14] and 1.0×10^{9} chemical reactions per second in each cell for a total of around 30 thousand billion billion chemical reactions in your body every second. That's 30 with 21 zeros after it. It's a big number, and all of this is happening inside of us regardless of whether we know it or not. This is our Infinite sustaining our finite. It is important that we see ourselves as miracles, as limitless and Infinite, because this mental perspective will allow us to participate in God's plan at the highest level possible.

It is important that we recognize that our body is functionally formed and that our mind is still forming and evolving. Therefore, the mind will need to be our area of focus for refinement throughout our life. This refinement is

---

[14] PLoS Biol, 2016 Aug; 148: e1002533,
Published online 2016 Aug 19. doi: 10.1371/journal.pbio.1002533

necessary because our brains have been hardwired over millions of years to sense trust or distrust in those around us for the purpose of survival.

When interacting with others, our brain senses whether we can trust the person we are with or not. If we can, we will open up, and if we can't, we will close down. If we sense trust, our prefrontal cortex (Ajna Chakra) is active, along with the "feel good" bio chemicals like dopamine, oxytocin, and endorphins, giving us a sense of well-being, enabling us to begin the journey of being in communion with another. In this state the two are co-creators of the conversation, which opens their minds up with a multiplier greater than two, allowing them to have intuition and foresight into Creation.[15] This is the most natural and safest way in which human beings are Infinitely connected.

On the other hand, if we sense distrust, we move to a different part of the brain—the amygdala (almond shaped, located in the limbic system, emotional processing center), which keeps us on guard so we can appropriately determine the level of reaction needed to keep us safe. Yes, this is our sympathetic nervous system at work helping us to not think but to react to the situation, which is to either fight, flight, or freeze. In this state, the body will release cortisol, epinephrine, and norepinephrine designed to help us win the battle in the moment, but this is not a state that we want to remain in for very long.

---

[15] Richard D. Glaser, PhD, "The Neuroscience of Conversations," *Psychology Today*, May 16, 2019

When we remain in environments (home, work, social, news) that are not trustworthy for extended periods of time, our distrust response fires repeatedly, and this chronic sympathetic state affects our health in numerous ways. All systems in our body are affected, including musculoskeletal, respiratory, cardiovascular, endocrine, gastrointestinal, nervous, and reproductive systems. Stress reduces our telomere length,[16] which shortens our lifespan and dampens the presence of our inner whisper, the Soul. Research suggests that chronic stress contributes to high blood pressure, promotes clotting in arteries, and causes brain changes that may contribute to anxiety, depression, and addiction.[17] When we are unable to avoid these environments, a daily practice of meditation will tone the brain to help us remain in a state of well-being, extending our life-span and reconnecting us to our Soul. It is critical that we understand this basic part of our nature, that we see that many of our struggles in life are not personal, but just necessary areas of refinement so that we can evolve into our next level of being.

---

[16] *Telomeres are tiny protective end caps on each of our chromosomes. They shorten as we age, and the shorter our telomere length, the shorter our expected lifespan and healthspan.

[17] Harvard Health Publishing, "Understanding the Stress Response," July 6, 2020,
https://www.health.harvard.edu/staying-healthy/understanding-the-stress-response

Chapter 2: Forming Your Finite

Understanding Our Immature Ego

Having Free Will means that we have total autonomy over our actions at all times. When our actions align perfectly with the Will of God, they originate from our mature ego mind, and when they don't align, they originate from our immature ego mind.

A mature ego mind longs for a deep connection with the Soul, because when we are connected with our Soul, our purpose perfectly aligns with the Collective Consciousness of the Universe. When our actions don't align with the Will of God, we are in our immature ego mind. When we are in this state, we are generally more self-serving, overly controlling, or out of control. We move in and out of these states throughout our day like a dance moving us in and out of function and dysfunction. We must become aware of our dance, so we can work to maintain a mature ego state, which allows us to participate at our highest state of existence.

It is easy to know when our immature ego mind is at work. It will try to convince us of the importance of who we are as an individual, that we fit in, and that we should please ourselves over others. It will build us up beyond who we are, which makes our fall back to reality frustrating, painful, and/or humiliating. The beauty of God is that She will turn even these blunders into good by

24

using them as learning points along our spiritual journey. It is important to reflect daily on the prevalence of our immature ego and redirect it, because if our immature ego state becomes chronic, it will pull us further away from our path of spiritual growth and increase the prevalence of behavioral (or mental) health conditions in our life.

To better understand the mental dynamics of our mind, imagine that our thoughts come from three inner voices: the child, the adult, and the elder. The mind is much more complex than this, but this analogy can help us to better understand the dynamics of our complex mental thinking. The child represents our desire to want things without thinking of the consequences and, at times, to impatiently want them. The adult represents our desire to control the child's ideas, many times through guilt, even when the child is right. And the elder represents our conscious, loving voice that is fully integrated into our Soul. The elder voice is always tied to our mature ego state, and the child and adult voices are always tied to our immature ego states.

There are two sides to the immature ego mind: an overdeveloped and underdeveloped ego mind. An *immature underdeveloped ego* is when the parent is overly controlling, causing the child to become insecure and afraid to act or make decisions, and an *immature overdeveloped ego* is when the child is overly controlling, many times wanting things (material, sex, power, etc.) that are only good for the ego self, not considering the effects of their actions on others.

One extremely dysfunctional part of an immature ego mind is how it perceives and manages its own pain and suffering. If the mind is unable to move through this state back into a state of peace, joy, and love, it will selfishly project its pain and suffering onto those around it. Often, those who live life this way imagine a God who causes pain. For centuries, many minds have perceived a pain-inflicting God, and to appease this God, many would sacrifice their precious possessions. However, this thought process was far from the truth, but a way for an immature ego mind to gain perceived control.

To move out of this state, we will have to embrace our fears and learn how to transform them, not transmit them into the world around us. To embrace your fear means to be humble, forgiving, compassionate, and loving. Through this process, we begin a journey of molding our ego into a mature state that helps us walk a spiritual life, a real life, a conscious life.

There is no need to make ourselves bigger than God expects. Finding our tiny selves, including our fears in this big world and infinitely large universe, might take a lifetime, but in the end will afford us more peace, joy, and love than our hearts and minds can imagine. Therefore, work to remove the illusion of pain and suffering, find your mature ego, and begin to live your life fully conscious!

Maturing Our Ego

Finding our mature ego is a natural part of living a Conscious life. This state is found when we are in balance, and it serves as a home base for evolving the mind away from our primitive states of survival and into states of Consciousness.

Ever since Adam and Eve, or the evolution of the brain to the point that it developed a conscience and could perceive God, we have been given the opportunity to participate in Creation. When our ego is mature, it sees the road ahead as a blessing, because the mind realizes the non-dual[18] world that it lives in, and when our ego is immature, life will seem to be a constant struggle, because it believes it lives in a dualistic[19] world.

When we maintain a mature ego, we have found a way to best manage the child and adult voices in our mind. If we can hold this state and have faith in God, God will share Her Creation with us. If we choose not to surrender, we will be shown temporary states of surrender in the humility we experience from our imperfect actions. If our imperfect actions become extreme, we may even hit "rock bottom," which forces the mind to surrender.

---

[18] *Non-dual* is a spiritual and religious concept where all things are infinitely interconnected in the universe, removing the illusion of the personal self. ("Nondualism," Wikipedia, https://en.wikipedia.org/wiki/Nondualism)
[19] *Dualism* is a belief that God is over there and I am over here.

If we hit "rock bottom," it feels personal, but it isn't. It is just the experience required for the mind to realize the benefits of falling into states of surrender. Knowing that life is non-dual allows us to see the endless opportunities for participating in God's Creation.

Finding our mature ego is as easy as finding stillness, for it is through our stillness that we are called into purposeful action. Without purposeful action, we are just plain sleepy and clumsy—"Forgive them. They know not what they do." Yes, even in our states of sleepiness, God will smile upon us, knowing that one day, through Her Grace, all will be one within us (body, mind, and Soul).

The voice of our purpose comes from the heart center (Anahata Chakra) and is projected into our body and mind. When we are conscious of this happening to us, we might find so much joy that a tear drips from the corner of our eyes. This is important because it is from these profound experiences that we witness the power of stillness and are driven to continue to find the Inner Voice of our Soul.

If we are ready to start the journey to the top of this mature ego mountain, we must first physically and mentally prepare the body and then have faith in the Soul to get us there. Climbing this mountain is divided into three stages. Stage one is physical preparation, stage two is love, and stage three is faith. These stages are sequential and get progressively more challenging from stage to stage.

Stage One – Physical Preparation

Stage one, physical preparation, is the easiest stage of maturing our ego and involves consuming healthy foods, moving the body in healthy ways, and getting proper restorative sleep. To do this, we have to weave healthy rhythms into our life so they are part of our daily routine. This is important because in the absence of healthy rhythms, our busy culture will suppress our ability to move through this stage successfully.

The first component of this stage is healthy food. Food is one of our most important medicines. Dietary advice and fads abound in society and can become overwhelming and contradictory. Keep it simple: eliminate ultra-processed foods, minimize added sugars, and eat a plant-rich diet full of the colors of the rainbow. Be intentional with your choices, and then begin to notice how your body feels.

To eat healthy, we need to consume micronutrients consisting of vitamins and minerals and macronutrients consisting of healthy proteins, carbohydrates, and fats. We need to become mini-scientists on understanding, finding, and eating these optimal foods to support the complex chemical reactions of the body. A good starting point each day is to drink at least half your body weight (lbs) in ounces of water, eat at least seven organic, non-GMO, plant-rich whole foods that comprise the colors of the rainbow, consume about half of your body weight (lbs) in grams of protein per day and include at least one serving of healthy fat three times per day.

The second component of the first stage is movement. The more we move, the healthier we become, and research has shown that getting to your target heart rate (220 minus your age times 0.8) for fourteen minutes each day will extend your life by seven years[20]. If you extend your workout time past fourteen minutes, you will begin to increase your metabolism's set point and burn fat.

The third component of this first stage is sleep. Sleep is a vital component of human life and essential for a person's health and well-being. Sleep occupies between 20 percent and 40 percent of the human day. It is often overlooked as a luxury; however, quality sleep is crucial to our health. Many restorative cellular functions occur during sleep. Stress and overstimulation with racing thoughts, to-do lists, and technology create disrupted sleep in a majority of people today. Sleep disorders have become a public health epidemic, with over 40 percent of us having reported some sleep disturbance in the past year.[21] Insomnia contributes to a host of medical conditions, including cancer, obesity, diabetes, depression, and hypertension. Sleep also affects our telomere length. Data shows that less than seven hours

---

[20] NIH, Does Physical Activity Increase Life Expectancy? ,https://www.ncbi.nlm.nih.gov/pmc/articles/PMC3395188/
[21] NIH, "What Are Sleep Deprivation and Deficiency?" https://www.nhlbi.nih.gov/health/sleep-deprivation

per night can prematurely shorten them and have a negative impact on our longevity.[22,23]

We have total control over this first stage (physical preparation), but it has to be something we want to do. You have to start with a *will* to do it. Then after the will is the *work* of integrating these positive changes into the rhythm of your life. If you are reading this book, there is an aspect of you that already wants to create positive change in your life. To accomplish this, you have to become a mini-scientist on how you personally are living and balancing the 4 Pillars of your health. You must surround yourself with experts and a community that helps you successfully navigate these positive changes. We have included a worksheet in the appendix to help you commit to monitoring these physical preparations daily (Breathe, Eat, Move, and Sleep Pillars). Once you have these basics, these necessities of life, down pretty well, you can start to move into stage two, self-love.

These next two stages get progressively more difficult to realize and maintain throughout life, therefore we have dedicated the following chapters of this book to help us

---

[22] Michael J. Breus, PhD, "How Sleep Affects Your Telomeres," Psychology Today, July 22, 2021, https://www.psychologytoday.com/us/blog/sleep-newzzz/202107/how-sleep-affects-your-telomeres

[23] Marta Jackowska et al., "Short Sleep Duration Is Associated with Shorter Telomere Length in Healthy Men: Findings from the Whitehall II Cohort Study," *PLoS One*, October 29, 2012, https://www.ncbi.nlm.nih.gov/pmc/articles/PMC3483149/#:~:text=Telomeres percent20were percent20on percent20average percent206,than percent207 percent20hours percent20per percent20night

dive deeper into the physical, quantum, and spiritual aspects of our body, mind, and Soul integration that will need to be in harmony, so that we may realized a joyful and loving Journey into Consciousness.

Stage Two – Self-Love

The second stage in maturing our ego is self-love. Once we master it, we will be called (initiated, awakened) into the Collection of Love (communion, love for all). When we love in this way, we turn on as an instrument of God. Once the instrument is turned on, the Soul will play the instrument in accord with the needs of Creation. This starts out slowly and builds in intensity until we are initiated into the next stage.

Stage Three – Faith

The third and final stage of maturing our ego—faith—is the hardest. It requires an unfettered ability to hold our deepest surrender, so that our Soul can project into us the needs of Creation. If the mind is toned and mature, one will experience bliss in aligning with the Collective Consciousness.

Understanding the complexities of the mind and working to direct and stabilize its function toward a mature ego state is the foundation of a Conscious life. Remember, it is more of a dance, and with time, we will become more coordinated, flowing, and graceful in how our dance leads us into Consciousness.

Chapter 3: Forming Your Infinite

Completely Significant and Completely Insignificant

We are called to awaken and see the gift that we are in the universe, to truly sit in awe of our greatness and infinite potential. Infinite because our full potential is not yet known.

How close is this infinite potential to your current purpose in life? Could it be as simple as moving through mundane tasks for most of the day and doing it over and over again? Possibly, if our actions are served from the Infinite, the Unseen, we will find much joy and love in doing so. For when we realize this vibration, we are "turned on" as an instrument of God's making, an instrument with infinite potential in the universe.

Meditation or contemplation is at the heart of this next level of our existence. Yes, we are all designed to do it, and each of us slip in and out of states of meditation multiple times a day, whether we are conscious of it or not. When we are ready to meditate consciously, there are a few nuances. We first have to learn to soften the ego and, more importantly, our immature ego mind. In the absence of this, our meditation often is filled with inappropriate thoughts of fear, lust, and/or control. Once we have mastered softening the ego, it gets thousands of times easier to sit in meditation. This is because in the absence of the ego, we are left with the whisper of our Soul, which feels like resting in our favorite comfy chair. When we find this state, it becomes our safe haven, our foundation for the mind to rest in as our heart explores the Collective Consciousness for our purpose today.

This Collective Consciousness is the intellectual collection of all things seen and Unseen. To scratch the surface of what the Collective Consciousness is in our life, let's start by exploring outward to the end of our universe and add up all the stars and then look at our one body and add up all the atoms . . . they are nearly the same number. Yes, there is an unimaginable universe outside us and one inside us ready to be explored, and our heart is resting right in the middle of this Collective Consciousness. Therefore, when we look into the vast expanse of the universe, we see that we are insignificant, but if our body hosts a universe within us, we must be totally significant at the same time.

Quantum Physics and the Unseen

With the latest discoveries in quantum physics, science is helping us to realize aspects of our Infinite. They have broken it down into three areas: matter, dark matter, and dark energy. Matter is composed of all things seen and measurable. This includes us, the earth, our solar system, our galaxy, and the culmination of all galaxies in the universe. The other two, dark matter and dark energy, are still a bit nebulous. Scientists know what dark matter isn't more than they know what it is, and imagine that dark energy could possibly have something to do with the expansion of space or, better yet, the creation of space within space. Their estimates are that our universe is composed of 4.9 percent matter, 26.8 percent dark matter, and 68.3 percent dark energy.[24] The point here is that the universe is mostly composed of dark matter and energy, and this is the stuff that fuels the Collective Consciousness.

Realizing the Infinite Potential Within You, Your Unseen

To consciously participate in the evolution of our human existence, one must understand the complexities of walking this path. It begins by understanding our individual journey and at the same time its complete integration with all things living. When the Flesh surrenders to the Soul, we begin to see and even feel our full potential as an instrument of Creation. In this moment, there is a Knowing that we are completely insignificant (immature ego surrenders) and fully significant (mature ego and purpose realized).

To evolve is to refine, to take what is crude/raw in us today and make it better, more useful, more purposeful for tomorrow. An immature ego mind sees what is crude as pain and suffering. To move beyond this we must turn on our refinery to process the pain individually, converting

---

[24] NASA, Dark Matter & Dark Energy, 2022, https://science.nasa.gov/universe/dark-matter-dark-energy/

it into beauty, into love. In this exact moment through our communion with all living things, the spirit, and therefore each Soul in the universe, sees our process of refinement and is able to utilize it within their evolutionary process of refinement with their physical form. When we refine even a little bit every day, we are walking a participatory life, a fully conscious life, a loving life!

This refinement process is infinitely complex, so to help us visualize and better understand the road ahead, yoga has broken it down into layers of our existence, the koshas, and the entry points for the Unseen into the seen through our body, the nadis (He is fully Divine and fully Human; "I and the Father are one"[25]). The Unseen has been awakening, revealing itself to all living things for millions of years. The reveal within humans will be unique person to person and be based on their current fund of knowledge, culture, and/or life experiences, which is why we have so many different terms for the Unseen across the globe, like the Holy Spirit, Prana, and Qi, just to name a few.

Buddhist, Hindu, Chinese beliefs, and yoga have documented this philosophy the most, with yoga terms like *koshas*, *nadis*, and *chakras* and Chinese terms like *meridians*. We will be focusing on the koshas, nadis, and chakras here because yoga is our area of expertise.

Kosha in Sanskrit means "sheath" and refers to the coverings over our Soul, moving us from the finite into the

---

[25] John 10:30

Infinite. Below, you will find their names and meanings. Of course, we are infinite beings, so I'm sure there are even more, but this will help us better understand and focus our work on refinement, making the road ahead easier to understand.

❖ Annamaya kosha, food sheath, Earth element (Anna)
❖ Pranamaya kosha, energy sheath, Water element (Prana)
❖ Manomaya kosha, mind sheath, Fire element (Manas)
❖ Vijnanamaya kosha, intellect/intuitive sheath, Air element (Vijnana)
❖ Anandamaya kosha, bliss sheath, Ether/Space element (Ananda)

Food Sheath

The food sheath is the easiest of all the koshas to understand and refine because it is a part of our finite world. When formed properly, it serves as a stable foundation from which all the other koshas safely rest upon. Remember the French quote, "You are what you eat."[26] Yes, when you fuel God's most complex living thing on this planet, the human body, with nutrient-rich whole

---

[26] "You are what you eat," is a translation of the French phrase "Dis-moi ce que tu manges, je te dirai ce que tu es" [Tell me what you eat and I will tell you what you are], written by French doctor Anthelme Brillat-Savarin in his book *Physiologie du Gout, ou Meditations de Gastronomie Transcendante*, 1826

foods from the Earth void of toxins and genetic manipulations, your body functions at its highest potential.

Healthy Eating is one of the Principle Pillars at OPT2LIV MEDICAL, because research shows a correlation between diet and altered gene expression, our epigenetics, that might have been a driving force in human evolution from chimpanzees.[27] If this is the case, the food we eat today will have a profound impact on the human race's evolution into our new states of Consciousness. Healthy eating is actually easy. We just need to recognize that it plays an important part in our path toward Consciousness and make it a priority. When we do this, it will make it easier to overcome our social pressures[28] and the convenience of eating unhealthy fast foods.[29]

Energy Sheath

This is the act of our Infinite Body (Soul) integrating into our finite body (food sheath). If the food we eat builds the

---

[27] Philip Hunter, "We Are What We Eat. The Link Between Diet, Evolution, and Non-Genetic Inheritance," NIH PubMed Central, *EMBO Rep.*, 2008 May; 9(5); 413-415. Doi: 10.1038/embor.2008.61, https://pubmed.ncbi.nlm.nih.gov/18451764/
[28] Social pressures can be a big obstacle on our journey toward Consciousness. Some examples include birthday cakes, chips, high-carb sugary foods, and libations.
[29] Our culture is so high paced and so over committed that it will be difficult to overcome the convenience of fast food, so it is important to educate yourself on the healthiest fast-foods with whole food options, like Chipotle, Bibibop, or Jimmy John's unwich.

body, then our Soul sustains our body and our Life. This is why when we die, the Life (Soul) leaves the body and the body remains.

Remember, it is impossible for us to totally understand how our Soul integrates into our physical body, but the following perspective for how yoga believes it happens has helped us to better grasp Its greatness, so that we can participate at a deeper level in Its integration.

In yoga philosophy, Unseen energy (Soul) enters into the body through points in the physical body called *nadis*. Even within yoga there are many different beliefs for how many nadis there are in the human body, but the one I have studied is the Hatha Yoga Pradipika, which believes there are 72,000 entry points or nadis in the human body that branch off into another 72,000 nadis all varying in size, with the largest ones called *chakras* that align the spine. Like meridians, nadis align with our nervous system, circulatory system, and organs, because these are our life force areas of the body, and prana is believed to be life force energy. There are three nadis that help us merge the chakras together, which are *ida*, *pingala*, and *sushumna*. These flow when the chakras are balanced, integrating our female and male energies (yin and yang) together to make us completely balanced and at our full potential, and in that instance in time, we are awakened, meaning that our body, mind, and Soul are fully integrated. Let it be known that this is the narrow path, the path less taken, but when we are able to achieve it consciously, we will be at our highest potential as a human being.

Chakras are vortices linking the Unseen and seen in the human body. From the Unseen side, this energy is Infinite, and from the seen side, they are massive energy centers designed by God to sustain our life across all aspects of our existence. These vortices spin like tops. When they are balanced, their spin is stationary and in control. From this state, they are able to express their highest refined potential. When they are unrefined, they are out of balance. In this state, they spin recklessly and are unpredictable and unstable. When they are unstable, our mind and body are unstable, and dis-ease and/or disease may develop.

Each chakra has a different vibration with a different effect on our physical body and mind. They each play a crucial role in helping us to form the mind into its highest state of ego maturity, and when the ego is matured, we align with our unique purpose in the world to fully participate with the Will of Creation.

The chakras have been a part of yoga philosophy for thousands of years. If you dive into the study of the chakras, you will find more divergence than convergence on the descriptions and definitions for each chakra, from color and shape to sound, smell, and so on. The association of the chakras with the colors of the rainbow was created in the 1970s by author Christopher Hill in his book, *Nuclear Evolution: Discovery of the Rainbow Body*.

41

This association of the chakras resonates with me more, so we will be building on this concept in the content to follow, but let your exploration of the chakras be organic, playful, childlike, fun, with no limitations. If Table 1 following highlights your base chakra (Muladhara) as red and you feel it to be a different color, then that is perfectly fine. Just know that your intimate discovery of these energy centers and your ability to balance them will help you fall into your full potential.

Table 1: Chakra Overview

Chakra Name	Focus Area	Color	Location	Kshetram	Unrefined State, Symptoms	Refined Potential
Muladhara, 1st	Male Energy	Red	Base of the spin, Root Chakra	N/A	Survival, fear, material possessions, fitting in	Seat of Kundalini, fearless, refined energy moves to bindu
Svadhisthana, 2nd		Orange	Root of sexual organs, Sacral Chakra	A little below the navel	Sexual desires, lust, perversion	Creative energy to do or create anything, unused energy moves to 4th chakra or above
Manipura, 3rd		Yellow	Navel, Solar Plexus Chakra	A little above the navel	Power, control, narcissism	An exemplary leader in the community, unused energy moves to 4th chakra or above
Anahata, 4th	Female Energy	Green	Heart, Heart Chakra	Center of chest	Projection of self-pain onto others, unstable emotions	Self love leads to loving others, joy, stable emotions
Vishuddha, 5th		Blue	Throat, Throat Charka	Throat pit	Lacking compassion, duality	In pure communion with all living things, non-dual thinking
Ajna, 6th		Indigo	Center of head	Center of eyebrows, 3rd Eye	Delusional, disoriented, lost	Intuitive, sees and feels the infinite in all around them
Sahasrara, 7th		Violet	Crown of head, Crown Chakra	N/A		Pure wisdom

This table shows: (1) the Name of the chakra, (2) the male and female energies' dominant Area of Focus, (3) the associated Color, (4) the Location along the spine, (5) the Chakras' projection point onto the front of the body, (6) typical Symptoms present if the Chakra is out of balance, (7) typical state realized when the Chakra is balanced.

To accelerate the rate of evolution, Creation has divided the work of refinement into two parts, yin and yang, or male and female energies (which is not to be confused with male and female genders) to reduce the load on each individual in their lifetime. Looking broadly down on society, it is clear that in today's world, female energies have naturally been graced with the upper four chakras and male energies the lower three chakras as their home base of work and refinement. The upper four are love, communion, intuition, and wisdom, and the lower three are survival, sex, and power. At a forty thousand–foot level, it is easy to see that there are opportunities for all humans to step closer to their full potential in this world, through balancing their male and female energies. Women tend to play the highest role in refining love on Earth and even realize an intensity for refinement of love after their first child. In general, men are designed for the hard work, the battles in life, and therefore are grounded in the chakras that need the most refinement on Earth today, the first three chakras.

Getting good at refining our energy will take time. It's like learning to ride a bike; we will first have to be willing to learn something new, which can be mysterious and scary at the same time, but with faith and hope we will successfully reach our desired endpoint. Initially our actions will appear fledgling and uncoordinated, but over time they will become functional or even highly functional as we get really good at our new skill.

At the height of mastering the Energy Sheath is the ability to self-heal or heal others, because when we flow with our Infinite, the body's potential for healing is infinite.

> Go; your faith has made you well.
> —Mark 10:52

> A cheerful heart is a good medicine, but a downcast spirit dries up the bones.
> —Proverbs 17:22

> Cure the sick who are there, and say to them, "The kingdom of God has come near to you."
> —Luke 10:9

It is from my personal experience of self-healing when I was ten years old that I realized and respected the importance of mastering the flow of our inner Infinite. Since our Souls are Infinite, we should expect each of our individual Spiritual experiences to be unique and different. It is our responsibility to keep an open and supporting mind to each other's unique journey toward the Spirit, so we can participate in the Spiritual growth of all human beings[30] on Earth.

---

[30] Vatican II, Declaration on the relation of the Church to non-Christian religions, Nostra Aetate, 1965

Mind Sheath

If we are purposefully on a path toward spiritual growth, we will spend our lifetime working to find and then maintain a mature ego state of mind. As a Catholic, I see this state as Christ Consciousness, but for others it might be the mind of Buddha, Krishna, Moses, Allah, etc. The point here is that we will have to take on a New Mind, a mind that sees through the illusion of separateness (dualism) and into the Collective Consciousness (non-dual), so that we can fully participate in Creation.

Intuitive Sheath

When our mind has shown that it can be mature, stable, and focused on the Will of God, the next layer of our existence awakens, and we are Graced with the ability to see into Creation through the Soul. This is the ability to be consciously in communion (interconnected) with all of Creation. It begins with being in communion with another human being and when we are ready, the ability to be in communion with all things.

We are all called to be in this state of communion with one another whether we know it or not. When we develop the ability to perceive the connection of communion with another, it becomes intuition, and in this moment we realize collective thinking, our ability to see beyond our own mind and into the Collective Consciousness of all minds. We generally think of this in our finite world as education, but this mode of learning is massively limited compared to the Infinite world of spiritual education, the Collective Consciousness.

As a living being, we are called to connect with all things living on this planet, and as a part of Creation, we are called to connect with all of Creation, living and material. We see this in ourselves when our heart tells us not to kill the spider. When we move this feeling from the heart and into the mind, we start to awaken this connection consciously.

Bliss Sheath

When this layer of our existence awakens, we will be blessed with the highest level of Grace an individual human being can receive. To achieve this state, we must move through all of the spiritual gates perfectly and be seated in a position to move beyond who we know ourselves to be as a human being and into a new super-conscious state of existence, like Jesus, Moses, Buddha, Krishna, and all the Saints, etc. As a Catholic, I know this to be true, because Jesus kept asking us to, "Follow Me." If we choose to walk this path, it will be our ultimate sacrifice, but in doing so we will afford the world a perfect example of what it means to be fully conscious.

At the onset of this sheath's awakening, God gives us a peek into this highest state of Consciousness so we can contemplate our level of readiness. It is like standing in a doorway right on the edge of the Grand Canyon, looking out into the unending vastness of the land to determine where the best place is to begin our hike, but instead of it being finite, it is Infinite. Moving through the doorway will be our ultimate sacrifice but allow us to achieve our highest state of existence as a Superhuman Being.

You will never see this Infinite with the mind, because it comes from a deeper Knowing in the heart.

Becoming Infinite

Becoming Infinite means being awake, fully conscious. To get to this point, we have to purposefully work a little bit every day to refine and evolve ourselves. When we are conscious, we see and embrace the journey ahead—every fault, wart, and blemish that we possess—and are willing to reform this aspect of who we are today for a better tomorrow. This type of work is easier to achieve when we have a daily practice, a rhythm woven into the fabric of our day that helps us chip away at our raw form so we can sculpt ourselves into God's masterpiece.

Chapter 4: Beginning the Journey

Finding Your Consciousness: Self-Examination

There are many opportunities in this life to explore the outside world, whether it is taking a walk, going to a family gathering, or finding an adventure to stimulate the mind. We could spend our whole life exploring our external world, gathering experiences and knowledge for the mind, and from this, find happiness. It is from these experiences of happiness that we sense an inner Knowing that there is much more to happiness, and it is from this Knowing that we begin our journey of self-examination. God has exposed us to these temporary states of happiness so we can discover the life-sustaining power of joy. For joy is the catalyst into our Consciousness.

Without a drive for self-examination, many people stumble through life like they are on a roller coaster ride consisting of temporary peaks of happiness followed by valleys of depression. This emotional roller coaster ride dampens our inner Knowing, slowing our Journey into Consciousness.

Everyone's Journey into Consciousness is different, and some will learn to explore their inner Self rather quickly, but most of us need a daily practice to open the doors to our inner Self. This daily practice may consist of meditation, contemplative prayer, or any other method by which an individual can begin to see their True Self (the Soul). Not unlike riding a bike, the first attempts at walking this path will be challenging and even test our ability to move through fear. When you want to accelerate your journey, it is ideal to have a teacher, an expert to show you the way. However, I guarantee you this: Once you learn how to journey inward, it will positively impact your life and the lives of the people around you forever, so what are you waiting for?

The journey inward is infinite and filled with more peace, joy, and love than one can even begin to imagine. This is why it is called KNOWING! Those who have been here clearly understand what I am saying, and those who haven't have an amazing opportunity awaiting them. This opportunity is not available to just a few; it is available to every human being, and it is by our design that it awaits our discovery.

This inward journey will allow one to realize an overwhelming sense of bliss. When one experiences this blissful state, there is an automatic association created in the mind that allows them to find this state again and again. With time, this Journey into Consciousness allows one to download enormous amounts of information, so that we can find our purpose and align with God's vision in this short life that we live. Once experienced, these blissful states will begin to replay during the day, helping us to stay focused and attuned to the true journey of our finite life.

God's vision is glorious, and with time, Her Vision of us as Her instrument will be realized. In the meantime, we have the opportunity to participate in Her continuous improvement process for the human form. This includes refining all the struggles, pain, and hardships that come with participating in the needed changes for today, so that the Glory of Her Creation may be realized tomorrow. God's forces are beyond our comprehension, and Her Will for change is beyond our control. These changes will occur to us either consciously or unconsciously, so why not find a way to align yourself with Her design and consciously live your life? We all are granted the opportunity to connect with God at this profound level. All we have to do is have Faith and Believe.

During the first steps into Consciousness, we are limited physiologically by the capacity of the organ of the brain to perceive all that is Real—"God's Dream." For example, if God's Creation is represented by every grain of sand on this Earth, then our brain has the capacity to realize one grain of sand at a time. In meditation, our goal is to concentrate on one grain of sand, like taking a still picture, to the point that we absorb deep into the grain of sand and become that which we concentrate on.

When you look at a beach, you know that it is a collection of sand tightly packed near each other, with one piece of sand touching many others. When we are able to master concentration and meditation, we will begin to have the capacity to move our concentration from one grain of sand to any of the other grains of sand touching the one we have been concentrating on. It is just like if you had two pictures in your hand with one stacked on top of the other. Once you are done looking at the top one, you remove it so you can see and begin to look (concentrate) at the second. This dynamic change in imagery when in a state of meditation is the ability to stream "God Consciousness." Again, this is only experienced after concentration and meditation have been mastered, somewhere past the Third Gate, because it takes a super-still mind to Truly see God's Consciousness unfettered or without illusion.

The hourglass is a perfect analogy for how our finite mind can stream God Consciousness. If we look at how hourglasses work, we know that sand starts at the top and is funneled down through a narrow gap, where just one grain of sand flows through at a time and then falls to the bottom. Think of the sand at the top as a collection of individual images that together represent a concept that we decided to meditate on, a collection of images that when viewed sequentially, allow us to better comprehend the concept, and the narrow gap, the capacity of our brain to process the images. The key to starting this process is to enter your meditation with a focus point (drishti, intention, etc.) and then surrender into the flow of Consciousness, like viewing an educational video. If one takes what is learned from their meditation and turns it into action, it is called *purpose*, and in this moment they are participating in the natural unfolding of God's Dream.

Our brain will never have the ability to fully comprehend the breadth and depth of God's Infinite Dream, but with meditation, we can begin to peer into aspects of Creation. The practice of yoga gives us the tools to find our Consciousness and, from this, to flow with the Collective Consciousness.

There is one step beyond this state where we transcend beyond the limitations of the brain completely (absence of "I," ego) to fully absorb into the entirety of God Consciousness, but this state is only accessible through complete mastery and the Grace of God.

Awakening your Consciousness: Building a Practice

According to William Harmless' book *Mystics*, ancient monks were compared to athletes. Monks were ascetics, and the Greek word *ascesis* was a sports term before it was a spiritual one. It meant "training," like Olympic athlete training, requiring the aspirant to renounce many things in order to find the highest level of athletic excellence. Where athletes focus on conditioning and disciplining the physical body, an ascetic focuses on conditioning and disciplining the mind.

Many challenges come up on the path of disciplining the mind. The move from physical to spiritual is natural but not easy. One has to successfully navigate through the forest of human desires and an immature ego so they can fall into their deepest surrender and rest in the hands of the Creator. From this state of surrender (meditation/contemplative prayer), the physical form, to include the mind, naturally opens up to receive the Infinite. This new awareness guides our actions (the Holy Spirit), our thoughts (Christ Consciousness), and our purpose (God the Father). When this state is achieved, one realizes what it means to be fully human and fully spiritual at the same time.

In order to hold this state, we have to master intimacy. Mastery of intimacy is the culmination of years of practice for holding the love of ourself and eventually the love of another. For many it started with the unconditional love of the mother or loved one, and from here, we mirrored this example in our relationship with ourself, our friends, our significant other, or our spouse. After years of practicing intimacy, we are called to hold this intimacy with the Creator. This relationship will change our life forever because it accelerates the flow of Consciousness and evolves our state of existence.

By the Grace of God, all human beings will one day realize this state of loving themself and others at all times—yes, at all times. In the meantime, we will need to work daily to overcome our powerful primitive instincts of survival that are wired deep within our DNA. Those who are already Conscious have been working on this journey for many thousands of years to get us to where we are today. Their preparation was driven by a personal practice to help them stretch and refine their physical, mental, and spiritual self on a daily basis.

We are creatures of habit, and research has shown this to be true. Our instinct is to take anything we do on a daily basis and make it as efficient and automatic as humanly possible. Research has shown that up to 90 percent of our day is habitual.[31] Each habit or rhythm that we have gets woven into our life until we have a new habit, and then over time, it, too, will get woven in. Once a rhythm becomes a part of our mental fabric, it is hardwired into the brain, making it very hard to unwire. This is being highlighted because our culture has us so busy that we rarely have margins in life to add one more thing, but this new rhythm will help you to see with new eyes the love of Creation all around you and how to participate in it.

To begin creating your practice, start simple. Have an intention to be still for a few minutes every day, literally just two minutes, and then let it grow naturally over time. Ideally, find a quiet and still place, leave your eyes open, focus on your breath, and keep your mind in the moment. It's that simple. What will happen naturally over time is that you will begin to fall into yourself, meaning that there will become a Knowing in the heart or an inner whisper in the mind that helps you to build a personal practice that accelerates your journey toward your highest spiritual potential. My journey started this way when I was ten years old and has evolved into the following practice

---

[31] Mark Buchanan, "Life, Why We Are All Creatures of Habit," NewScientist, July 4, 2007, https://www.newscientist.com/article/mg19526111-700-why-we-are-all-creatures-of-habit/

summary. The detailed version can be found in the appendix.

This practice serves as a means to prepare my body and mind to flow with the Spirit and God's Infinite Grace:

I.   Preparation, light candle
II. Centering, find stillness
III. Moving Meditation, concentration, remove tension
IV. Reiki, remove energy blockages
V.   Kriya, cleanse the body
VI. Pranayama, regulate energy
VII. Still Meditation/Contemplation

If you would like a virtual guide to help you build or rekindle your practice, please goto www.opt2livcourses.com and choose our OPT2CHANGE 21 Day Wellness Program.

Refining Your Consciousness, Becoming Fearless

When we are on a pilgrimage toward total Consciousness, we will be challenged with passing through narrow gates along our journey of Enlightenment.

> Enter through the narrow gate; for the gate is wide and the road broad that leads to destruction, and those who enter through it are many.
> —Matthew 7:13

These gates are sequential and build on each other. We are only able to pass through a gate once we have proven our worthiness. Until then, we will wait outside the gate working to refine ourselves into a more acceptable state of being. The gates operate more on a pass/fail scale, which means there are some that get through with a perfect A while others squeeze by with a C-. This is important to note because a higher grade is associated with more work upfront but with less perceived suffering down the road.

The First Gate, Finding Love

In the first part of life (birth to seven years), by the Grace of God, we are shown Her Glory, so that we can see and desire a journey toward Love. For many, this Grace flows in their finite world through the example of their parents' love. If this example isn't present physically, it flows in as a whisper from one's Infinite Soul. The intensity of this Grace is present in our life until a model of Love is imprinted in our mind forever. This imprint only occurs after the mind accepts or surrenders to God's Grace. This is our first initiation into a spiritual life and is our First Gate. It is important to note that God's example of Love is perfect and complete, but that our interpretation of this perfect love, in the finite mind, will be limited by our body's current state of health and well-being, causing all human imprints of love to be unique and different person to person.

The Second Gate, Mental Control

Our next stage in life, years eight to fourteen years, seems to be very complex and challenging, because this is a time when our body changes both physically and emotionally at the same time. On the physical side, male and female hormones get created and released to start the process of puberty, while at the same time our emotions become more driven by powerful instincts for survival and intimacy. This is the Second Gate, the gate of emotional control, our ability to stay contemplative and conscious amidst physical and emotional chaos.

If our physical chaos (hormones) are wired into our DNA and therefore out of our control, and our emotional chaos is directly related to our environment and in our control, it will be vitally important to become mini-scientists for how hormones impact our well-being. Think of hormones as emotional light switches that get turned Off and On based on our environment, and then study your environment, the interactions with other people, the food you eat, and the exposure to toxins, and remove or change the areas that are not benefitting your quality of life.

This is why establishing a healthy baseline for love and morality during the first stage of life is so important. In the absence of this baseline, it is easier for our emotional states to become chronically out of balance, leading us into unnecessary states of fear, anxiety, instability, gluttony, lust, and individualism.

Be patient with yourself and know that any undesirable mental states that were wired into the brain over time will be unwired once we find more joy-filled life habits. This process of change is extremely complicated, so it will take awareness, focus, and discipline to successfully navigate, but in the end, it is the process that navigates you through the second gate.

The Third Gate, Self-Love

The following two gates are still sequential, but not tied to changes in our physiological time clock like the first two.

The third gate will test our ability to find comfort in who we are and how we are called to serve in our life (purpose). It is our ability to accept all that we are in every moment in time, our successes and our faults, and maybe even more so our faults.

If you are already on your spiritual journey, then you know there is much work to do as individuals and in society before we are all at our endpoint as superhumans on this planet. With this at the forefront of our mind, it is clear that we are called to see our faults, embrace them, and then work to refine what we know is imperfect, allowing us to take one step closer to the positive change that we are called to be in this world.

To step past this gate, we have to move through our powerful survival instincts to 1) fit into society (back in the

59

day, fitting in meant staying alive), 2) eat (finding food to survive), and 3) procreate (necessary for sustaining human life). Unconscious people react to these instincts at home, at work, or with friends on a daily basis, and can get stuck here, never making it through the spiritual gate of self-acceptance and purpose.

When you look out into a field filled with birds and one takes off, the majority of the birds will take flight with only a few remaining. Are you the few or the many? It's probably a little of both, but the goal is to move more toward the few, because in doing so, you move closer to being conscious with your instinctive reactions to life.

To do this, we need to understand our physiology on a deeper level so we can see that our struggle to move through this gate is more dependent on our ability to manage our innate physiological responses to the world around us than it is that we do not want to find our purpose in life. When we look at it this way, we see that the struggle is not personal; it is just a part of our physiology that we need to refine and mold into a higher-functioning state.

In the mid-part of the brain is our limbic system. This is our "bells and whistles" area of the brain, which constantly monitors the world around us, making sure we are safe. It comprises the amygdala, responsible for our emotions, and the hippocampus, responsible for our memories. Both help us to unconsciously respond to our environment by releasing dopamine into the brain as a reward when we do something perceived to be correct. Looking inside the brain, we would see neurons, our brain cells, and neurotransmitters (chemical messengers) that send signals back and forth between the brain cells. Dopamine is one of many neurotransmitters that, when released, causes us to feel contentment and euphoria.

Functionally, dopamine gets released so we can find healthy life rhythms for how we interact every day in life, like knowing when to eat, how often to move, when to sleep, and how often we should have sex. For many, this chemical gets out of balance, and when it is out of balance, it creates addictive responses for how we eat, how often we move, when we sleep, and even how often we want to have sex. It is also the chemical that gets released when we consume drugs, and we all know or have known how challenging it can be to overcome these habits when out of balance. Therefore, it will take a considerable amount of awareness, discipline, and focus to maintain balance in the brain's dopamine response so we can move through this gate. This is what many of the lifestyle-altering programs like Exodus 90, Hard 75, or strict diets have the potential to show us.

Once we find this balance, we find healthy contentment. Healthy contentment is self-love, and self-love leads to relaxation or surrender. A surrendered self will always find its purpose, because in this state we see and operate from the Soul's whisper deep within. This is the state we need to find and hold to move through the third gate. Once we pass through, we will never go back, because we are now molded into a "New Form." We become "Awakened," or some call it "Born Again," and will forever see the world through a "New Lens."

Fourth Gate, Communion

Many have heard the phrase, "Again, [amen,] I say to you, if two of you agree on earth about anything for which they are to pray, it shall be granted to them by my heavenly Father. For where two or three are gathered together in my name, there am I in the midst of them."[32] Our natural ability as instruments of God to connect at an unseen level is our ability to be in communion with one another, and when the day comes that all human beings on this planet have moved through this gate, we *will* change the face of the earth.

Once we have passed through the third gate, God sees that we are prepared to participate at a higher level in the Collective Consciousness of planet Earth and the universe, because we have shown that we can refine our own faults into good and therefore are able to do the same for others in an unseen way. The first step in preparing to move through this gate is to attain and sustain our mental health and stability. In the absence of this level of mental health, we will become mentally exhausted and unstable, especially if we fall back through our lower gates.

---

[32] Matthew 18:19-20 NABRE

Take, for instance, the challenges in making positive change in our own life, and then multiply it times every unseen connection of communion that we have with others. When this happens, you can imagine that for our own health and safety, there comes a point where if the work becomes too challenging, we may need to reset ourself by consciously disconnecting all of our connections of communion, giving them back to God, and then grounding into nature or Mother Earth until our mind regains the mental health needed to again serve at this level of spiritual participation.

Mothers know this connection more than anyone, because they automatically pass through the fourth gate during their forty weeks of pregnancy to fall into communion with their child inside their body. This is one of the reasons why women's spiritual set point is naturally higher than men's and that men, on average, will need to be more vigilant and more disciplined to achieve the same level of spiritual participation as women. Maybe this is also one of the reasons why the twelve apostles were men and not women, because men have a longer road of spiritual growth ahead of them.

Once God sees that we have the physical and spiritual purity to operate at this level, we pass through this gate and begin to serve at a higher level of spiritual participation. This road less traveled always goes uphill at an ever-increasing rate. Therefore, on the other side of this gate, we need to be prepared to witness some of our most challenging spiritual times in life yet to come. The sixteenth-century Spanish mystic, St. John of the Cross, called it the Dark Night of the Soul, a time of mental disorientation and spiritual purification.[33] Once we realize that this is more of a gift and less of a personal attack on us, that God has chosen us as worthy to participate in the unseen spiritual molding of others, it will make our journey toward reorientation and purification a natural rhythm in our life. This happens because our spiritual growth is less linear and more oscillating at an increasing rate.

Living a simple life reduces the propensity of spiritual oscillations, lightening the load along the spiritual path less traveled. This simple life can be seen in mystics, monks, sisters, and clergy and during a person's healthy last years of life, giving them the potential to serve at a safer and higher capacity than householders. The householder path is the path of anyone who chooses to be in a relationship or marry and have children. Anyone on this path knows the innate dynamics of family life that at times can create tremendous oscillations in life, challenging both our physical and spiritual journeys.

When the mind becomes settled amidst our service of communion with others within this gate, we will have moved out of our fledgling state and into our highest spiritual state of maturity for this gate. Finding this state means that we have found comfort in the non-dual universe that we live in and are fully ready to participate in God's plan for us.

---

[33] "Dark Night of the Soul," Wikipedia, https://en.wikipedia.org/wiki/Dark_Night_of_the_Soul

Fifth Gate, Total Consciousness

If we have moved through the fourth gate successfully and have a personal daily practice of meditation, there may become a point that by the Grace of God only, we are given the gift of sight into Her Creation. This experience is profound, reorienting the mind so that we can see even more clearly into the Glory of Creation. There are two opportunities during this gate: the first is that we choose to stand in the doorway and gaze into Creation, and the second is that we pass through the doorway to participate at an even higher level in Creation.

Even if we choose to just stand in the doorway of Creation, it will positively impact our life forever, giving us a new lens for looking into the world around us. If God sees you worthy, you will be asked to serve at the next level of participation. This road ahead will be shown to you, so that you can contemplate if your Will is ready to become Superhuman, Saintly, and operate at the highest level of human existence. Passing through this gate will change all aspects of who we know ourself to be today, our finite, our body and mind, our Infinite Soul, and even how our Infinite moves into our finite (chakras). To determine our path, we will need time to discern with a contemplative mind, so that we can see clearly if our Will is strong enough to navigate this highest level of spiritual existence.

Whoever wishes to come after me must deny himself, take up his cross, and follow me. For whoever wishes to save his life will lose it, but whoever loses his life for my sake will find it.
—Matthew 16:24-26

Yes, you will have to be Willing to give up everything to find this highest state. If you are ready, please take the leap, for this is who we are called to be. Our examples are Jesus, Buddha, Krishna, and all the Saints.

Chapter 5: Conclusion

By the Grace of God each day more and more people are being shown The Journey into Consciousness. The journey begins when one chooses to soften their little self, the immature ego, so that their big Self, the Infinite Soul, can be realized. When this awakening of our Self occurs we are initiated into the Journey of Consciousness and presented with a New Mind, a mind of communion with all that leads us into inner peace, joy, and love. This Journey into Consciousness is in full stride when we have found comfort in our inner whisper and have released the significance of control, selfish desires and personal gain.

In order to stay on our Journey into Consciousness we will have to embrace the responsibilities that come with maintaining the minds' new evolved state. It will require a lifetime commitment of tuning and refining the mind individually and collectively. Our individual journey might include a daily meditation practice, with reflection that supports a playful willingness to surrender to Self (Soul), allowing us to explore our mind's new evolved perspectives. The collective journey comprises our initiation of communion with all living things and a discovery of like minded people to safely evolve our Journey into Consciousness.

If you are reading this then you have been called to be the first of few examples for others to follow. Have Faith that your willingness to Journey into Consciousness will positively impact your life and be a positive change for

Life on Earth. The day will come when all living things on this planet will live in harmony and by your will and dedication today it will be realized even sooner. Dare to be your highest potential. Dare to be a New World Explorer. Dare to be a positive Change in the World.

Part II: A Culmination of Conscious Thoughts

by Eric Banter

Chapter 6: Conscious Thoughts

How to Use These Conscious Thoughts

At the end of my morning meditations, I enjoy sitting and writing the thoughts still in my head. This practice began back in 2010 and continues today as a way for me to see into Consciousness.

Although there are many ways to use these muses to support your Journey into Consciousness, the following is a practice to consider.

Find a quiet time during the day to sit in stillness. Your stillness will bring you into the moment reducing the propensity of the mind to wander into the future or into the past. Now take slow deep steady breaths to relax the body and mind. If you feel a little anxious then allow your exhale to be longer than your inhale for at least two minutes (2 to 1 Breathing). Concentrate on the integration of your body, mind, and Soul, for it is from this state that we can witness the edges of Consciousness.

Now read a Conscious Thought and relax even further into stillness. If you are new at this keep your eyes open during your stillness and with time you might choose to close them. Now become an observer of your thoughts and allow them to flow as if they were in a river, meaning that their intensity diminishes second by second. At this time it is important to keep the flow going, so that you do not ruminate on just one thought. After a minute or two, begin to notice the theme of your thoughts and follow them. Ask yourself, "Are the thoughts collective or personal in nature? Are they for my viewing pleasure or a call for personal change? Where are the thoughts guiding me?". If the mind remains Conscious you will see the positive side of your thoughts, and if the mind moves away from Consciousness and into primitive thinking, you will find yourself controlling the thoughts, taking them personal, and ultimately seeing the negative side of the thoughts. If you notice your mind moving negatively just gently nudge it back into Consciousness and over time you will naturally see the positive side of life and your place in it, your purpose.

However you choose to use these muses, maintain a playful, curious, and compassionate mind for this will keep the primitive immature ego mind at bay, giving your Conscious mind unfettered room to roam, grow and evolve.

1- Additive Actions

The manifestation of Creation is patiently moving life toward a Pure Love Consciousness over time. In the beginning, all living things must have a will to live and survive. This initial form of thinking will naturally cause us to think individually. In this moment of life, the one is seen to be more important than the whole. This is perfect for the initial stages of life but is not the endpoint. In our next stage of life, we sense Consciousness, the Unseen Whisper within us, guiding us beyond the binary reactions of our instincts and into actions of pure love. From here our Consciousness sees the communion of the whole and the importance of our full surrender to the Grace of God, so that all of our actions are additive to God's Will and Creation.

2- Today Is a New Day

When we are in survival mode, we mainly just think of ourselves. When we are conscious and in communion with all things, we see the Glory of God's Creation and us within It. How do you know if you are in survival or conscious communion mode? When we take things personally, we are in survival mode, and when it feels like we are flowing with the world around us or when life seems effortless, we are in communion. Now, my buddy Jesus, as the Son of God, was born into this World in full communion with all things. It was from this communion and His state of All Knowing that his purpose was clear, to selflessly share His loving actions and acts of kindness with us to show us "The Way." Yes, He was way beyond taking things personally, because from His state of communion, He knew that humans were still being created. He knew that we were more clumsy, like a child learning to walk, than we were fully realized as an instrument of God.

Luke 23:34: Jesus said, "Father, forgive them, for they do not know what they are doing."

So the next time you start to take things personally, open your heart and mind to see yourself in communion with all, and from this vantage point find forgiveness and patience today, for our future is a world full of loving people.

Matthew 26: But Jesus looked at them and said to them, "With men this is impossible, but with God all things are possible."

Be Glad, Believe, and have Faith that today is a step toward the Glory of God!

3- Preparing the Brain for the Future of Mankind

Our brain is a very complex organ. It plays an integral part in controlling our organs, thoughts, memory, speech, and movements.[34] It has evolved over hundreds of thousands of years, getting us to where we are today, but there is

---

[34] "What Is the Physical Composition of the Human Brain?" Healthline, April 8, 2019, https://www.healthline.com/health/is-the-brain-a-muscle

still room to grow. If we think of the brain as a supercomputer, which it is, and measure how it operates in the same way, then we find that an immense amount of communication takes place between the body and the brain, helping us to evaluate the environment that surrounds us at any moment. This makes sense from an evolutionary standpoint, because an accurate determination of our environment allowed us to stay away from the edge of the cliff, run from the tiger, and eat the right food, keeping us alive to enjoy our life for as long as possible. Knowing this, we can also see why yoga is such an effective tool to help us calm the mind and begin to learn the art of removing the senses (Pratyahara), to quiet the unnecessary sensory chatter of our survival instincts. I don't know where you live, but in Indiana, we don't have any tigers :-), so, yes, it is definitely time for Hoosiers to move out of survival mode :-). The less chatter, the more room to be conscious. To make my point clear, science has now determined that the load on the mind from our senses can be upwards of eleven million bits per second, whereas consciously reading a book takes about fifty bits per second.[35] You probably see the point, but to make sure that you do, our brains are mostly geared for survival, not Consciousness . . . yet. This is why it is so important to find time every day or multiple times every day to "Be Still and Know God."[36] This tones the brain to be ready and able when you truly need to be conscious. If everyone on this Earth was on this journey, we would find

[35] "Application of Information Theory," Britannica.com, https://www.britannica.com/science/information-theory/Applications-of-information-theory
[36] Psalm 46:10

ourselves in a consciously loving environment. In the meantime, part of our job is to be patient, find our own practice for being still, and be a loving example for others to see.

4- The Good in Evil

It is interesting to watch the emotion that gets stirred up when people start to talk about the devil or evil acts from other people. Is this emotion tied to justice and our desire to want to control the actions of others, or is it our scapegoat for an inability to control ourselves? It's probably a little bit of all of this. Yes, on a personal level there is a force that is opposite peace, joy, and love in the world, and it usually looks like fear, lust, greed, hatred, pain, and/or suffering. Could it be that these more negative experiences in life are a training ground for human beings to evolve into a Superhuman state? If you believe in Moses, Jesus, Buddha, or Krishna, then you already know that this is true, for it is only through our ability to refine our own and others' pain and suffering that we walk a journey into sainthood. The easiest way to begin the journey is to graduate from our personal or individual work of Consciousness into the communal work of Consciousness. Once we get initiated into communal work, it is imperative that we get comfortable with being uncomfortable or that we find a total state of surrender, because the work ahead will be done unto us.

5- Complementary Relationships

When each person in a relationship spends much of their energy in a day supporting and filling the voids of the other, you will find a complementary relationship, one filled with much joy and love. If one or both in a relationship spend more time satisfying themselves over their partner, then with time, the presence of joy and love in the relationship diminishes. The feelings of joy and love are God's reward to an individual for participating in Creation. It is designed to be a mountaintop experience, and for many, this could happen multiple times a day. During this experience, time stands still and we fall into a state of contemplation or total surrender, which equals total participation in God's Will. God has designed this experience to be profound, so that we are encouraged to find it again. When we begin our descent from this mountaintop experience, we move into the working part of maintaining our relationships. During this time, we need to be observant, intuitive, and caring toward the other, so that we can see the best way to complement our partner, and then work selflessly toward filling their voids. This is the essence of pure communion. Our training started with our mother, then our family and friends. When we prove competency in these relationships, God presents our spouse, which will prove to be more dynamic, more unpredictable, and more humbling, but when done selflessly, infinitely rewarding. It is imperative that we Give to Receive, not Give only if we Receive. This can be extremely difficult for an immature ego. Therefore the work for all humans in relationships is to recognize the state of their ego and move it as well as possible toward a state of maturity. For the most part, our immature ego is prevalent when we are in survival mode, and our mature ego is present when we are conscious beings. By the Grace of God we are all on a path of Consciousness, but if you want to accelerate the journey, you will need a practice that allows you to fall into your essence (Soul) daily, for a mature mind, a Christ Conscious Mind, can only come from our Soul, and the Soul from the Spirit.

6- Bonds of Creation

If bringing two atoms together to make a molecule is called *chemistry*, then bringing two people together to make a marriage is called *communion*. When we open our minds up to see the non-dual world that God is Creating, it is clear that all things are created to complement one another, and from this, to bring newness into the world. We have all heard the phrase from physiologist Robert Francis Winch, "opposites attract," from his study of spouses, where he found that what people are really looking for in a life partner is someone who complements their personality.[37] To find this type of spouse is to find communion. When we are in communion, we extend ourselves way beyond the basic laws of math, where 1 +

[37] Robert Francis Winch, "The Theory of Complementary Needs in Mate-Selection: Final Results on the Test of the General Hypothesis," *American Sociological* Review, Vol. 20, No. 5 (Oct., 1955), pp. 552-555 (4 pages)
Published By: American Sociological Association,
https://doi.org/10.2307/2092563

$1 = 2$, and begin to participate in the Unseen realm where $1 + 1 =$ infinity, the boundless essence of God's Creation.

By the Grace of God, we are put together to make something New. It is not personal; it is for Creation, not dissimilar to how God has brought hydrogen and oxygen together to make water. When God brings things together, there is a massive amount of unseen energy entering into this seen world, and for conscious beings, it feels magical or euphoric. This is God's wedding gift to the couple.

Like how a mother cares for her child until it becomes an adult, God cares for all of Her bonds in Creation until they have matured. This graduation is important so that each individual can experience what it takes to hold God's bond of communion on their own. This is the yin and yang, the give and take, and the art of holding your spouse's opposite, for it is through this action that we fully participate in the Will of God.

7- Faith or Fear

Faith is the home base for saints, and fear is the home base for animals. Fear is driven by the innate biology of all living things to want to survive. Our *amygdala*, an almond-shaped set of nuclei in the center of the brain, is designed to detect the emotional importance of the stimuli, and then the *hippocampus*, which is closely connected to the amygdala, and the *prefrontal cortex*, the part of the brain that actually looks like a brain, interpret and perceive the threat to determine the next steps. They help us decide whether we should stay calm (the parasympathetic mode of the nervous system) or fight, flight, or freeze (sympathetic mode of the nervous system). The point here is if we want to move away from a mind full of fear and into a mind full of Faith, we will have to find ways to tone how our brain reacts to the environment around us or even change our environment.

Our environment today is much more dynamic than it was one hundred years ago. Back in the day, the nuances in our environment for the brain to navigate were a cliff, another human, or maybe an animal, but today the complexities of our environment are too great and, frankly, very confusing to our mind, which we see in the increasing rate of behavioral health conditions at all ages but even more so with our younger generation. This mental confusion is directly related to how often in a day we listen to the radio, watch TV, get on the internet, check emails, or use the cell phone. Our brain will perceive each of these as a new environment and will work to determine if there is a threat. If it believes you are in danger, even though you are just watching the news, it will proceed through the steps of setting off the alarms, putting you in fight, flight or freeze mode, dropping your IQ by 50 percent, and keeping you there for up to four hours until the threat has been avoided and your hormones have been reabsorbed or removed from the body. This is way too costly to do on a repetitive basis, which is why you need to establish an electronic hygiene protocol to give your brain a break.

Here are a few things we have done in our family: stopped watching the news, rarely listen to the radio, spend more time in nature or outside, and smile as often as possible, so that you're not perceived as a threat to other people. Once we do this, we will have more time in our day to focus on Faith. This is our next step in fully participating in Creation as the most complex living thing on the planet. You are a gift and a blessing; find a way to be your best today!

8- Embracing Humility

We have to become patient with ourself as we venture deeper into becoming fully Conscious. There is a basic theme for walking the narrow path: one has to have the ability to see through their personal suffering and the collective suffering in the world. From this lens, it is easier to see God, Consciousness. When we rest in Consciousness, we realize the dichotomy between where we are now and where we are called to be. To rest in this Knowing is called humility, our ability to fully see and accept ourself and the world around us. This work of seeing where we are now and where we are called to be, and from it refining and remolding ourself to become the best version of ourself, should be slow, meticulous, and contemplative. Embracing these qualities provides a higher probability of sustainable change. Otherwise, our life usually feels more like three steps forward and two steps back over and over again. During these struggles, if we don't have humility, we will fall off the narrow path.

Yes, gradual change is sustainable change, and sustainable positive change changes the world.

9- Shaktipat Kundalini

Although we look mostly finite, with a body, skin, hair, eyes, etc., this is just a tiny piece of who we really are. If we really looked at our whole existence, we would see that we mostly consist of Infinite stuff with a little bit of finite stuff. Many will go through life seeing only their finite with occasional glimpses of their Infinite, like the standing still of time when we hold a baby, watch the sun rise, or see a flock of birds take flight. There is a Knowing during these times, deep within, that there is much more to the world around us. We feel a sense of peace that leads us to joy and love, and when these states of Consciousness are invoked in the body, we brush up against our Infinite for a moment in time.

How important is this Infinite? Unknown to us, it sustains us thousands of times more than the food we eat, the water we drink, and the air we breathe. It is our True life-sustaining substance, our healing faculty, our total Consciousness, and it flows through every aspect of our physical body. This flow is directly related to our ability to soften, to relax, to surrender. Think of it this way: if our finite body was the light bulb, then our Infinite would be the electricity. Together, they have the capacity to light up a room. The switch that controls the flow has two modes: OFF is when we are holding tension or dis-ease, and ON is when we soften, relax, or surrender.

This flow mostly originates from our Infinite or our Soul, but it can also flow from another. This can be called many things, but in my lineage of yoga, it is referred to as Shaktipat Kundalini. This operates only from the Grace of God and can never be forced, but has the ability to help another realize what it feels like to flow with their Infinite, increasing the number of fully awakened human beings in the world.

10- Dialing in Your Ego

To find the mature side of our ego is to find our purpose. Many times we associate our ego with the faulty side of ourselves, the side that produces actions that are not additive to the world around us. This occurs when we are not dialed into the home base that God has called us to fall into, our purpose. To simplify this infinitely complex unseen dynamic in our life, it would look like a parabola, where the horizontal axis represents the presence of ego ("I"), and the vertical axis represents the additive effect of our ego actions.

To better understand this, let's break our horizontal line into three sections. At the leading edge of the line is an under-defined ego (immature state), in the middle a balanced ego (mature state), and at the far edge an over-developed ego (immature state). We all cycle through aspects of all three throughout our day, but are called to dial in and hold the mature state for as long as possible. This is directly related to our ability to find and hold our Conscious mind, our Soul, because from here we realize our purpose in the moment, maximizing the positive effects of our actions in the world around us. In this state, our parabola looks like a really tall, narrow bell, void of our immature ego states and infinitely full of our mature ego mind and purposeful actions[38].

11- Stabilizing Your Intuitive Sense

Our brain today is one of the most complex living organs on this planet. It has evolved over time from a primitive binary processor to help us safely react to our environment, to a massively complex processor that organizes our memories, perceives our environment, plans our future, and much more. There is so much in the "much more" that it would take a lifetime to parse through it all, so let's just look at a couple of areas.

One that we all know well is our "gut feeling" faculty that helps us sense if the person we are standing next to is good or bad. This isn't tied to our memories or basic senses, but rather comes from a feeling deep within us. It seems like our animal friends use this faculty often. The other one that we should highlight is our intuitive faculty. This faculty allows us to see beyond our own thoughts into all thoughts, into Consciousness. This faculty is turned on by the Grace of God only after one has proven the ability to properly refine and process their own thoughts. Initially, when this graduation occurs, it is very disorienting to the individual, because you have to learn

---

[38] See Appendix topic, A Journey Toward the Unseen

which thoughts are yours and which ones aren't, or you will question yourself: "Why am I thinking this? Is there something wrong with me?" "Why am I having inappropriate thoughts?" If our ego isn't matured fully, then we can get lost in this new state of confusion. If this is the case, it is important to ground yourself to remove the confusion. You can ground out by taking a walk in the woods or hugging a tree for more than ten seconds. But with time, like a child learning to walk, we become less clumsy and are able to utilize this new faculty to finely perceive and participate at the highest level in the world, Consciousness.

12- Renew the Face of the Earth

At one point in our life, there becomes a Knowing that there is more to life than what we see. This creates an inner desire to explore our new Knowing. When our exploring becomes a permanent rhythm in life, then our Knowing becomes clearer, and its comfort can be seen and felt on many levels. Over time, a pathway is formed, allowing us to easily return to our new Knowing for restoration of the physical body and renewal of the mind. Once your personal pathway is formed, you will be called to help others to find their Knowing and personal pathway. This happens in two ways: one is in the seen through our example in life, and the other is in the Unseen through our transmittal of Spiritual Energy, Shaktipat Kundalini. When it comes to the Unseen, there isn't much that you have to do, because it is being done unto you. Follow your Knowings, have a practice, fall into Holiness, and surrender to the works of God all around you. Then know that your conscious work will impact the next seven generations of people and renew the face of the Earth!

13- Feeling the Flow

We perceive the physical world around us with our mind and our senses. From here, our mind takes over to assimilate our seen, and safely navigates our body one step at a time through time and space. This is its primitive function. Only once the mind realizes that it is safe will it venture out of this unconscious state into Consciousness. For this to happen, the mind takes on a new sense, allowing us to perceive and connect with the Unseen. From the onset, we begin to perceive the infinite flow of the seen and Unseen all around us and begin to feel and believe that all is one and one is all. This is the birth of our non-dual mind. Once we taste this side of reality, our mind can never go back, because the image of the Infinite is imprinted deep within our existence for the rest of our physical life. This state of metanoia opens our eyes to the importance of our actions in the physical realm, causing our mind to seek the depths of our purpose in life. Once we have the Infinite planted deep within and our mind aligned with our purpose in life, we are able to rest in pure joy and love, for we have blossomed into our highest potential.

14- Inward Gazing

The more comfortable we are at going inward to gaze at our raw self, and from this inward Knowing willing to step closer to our optimal state as an instrument of God, the quicker we are able to achieve our own little states of Holiness. It is truly not necessary to move mountains, build an arc, or heal lepers in our life. Our work should focus on simple daily actions that move the collection of all beings toward a union of love. This inward journey should start by establishing and then getting comfortable with a personal practice of prayer, meditation, or contemplation. During these states of relaxation and stillness, the mind naturally goes inward to review thoughts and memories. In this first level of mental review, the mind asks the question, "Are we safe?" If there is even just one "yes" anywhere in the mind, the mind remains here until it can resolve the question. This is why it is so important to resolve past traumas and truly forgive those who have inflicted physical and mental pain and suffering in our life, or we will become stuck and never reach our full potential. When we have resolved the first question, we ask the second question, "Who should we love or serve?" We stay here scanning our mind and physical surroundings until we have identified our connection(s), then work to build a loving relationship. If this loving connection disengages and we become hurt, we move back to ask the first question, "Are we safe?" and remain here until this question is resolved. If our immature ego hangs on to a need to control others or even the dynamics of life, we will remain in a perpetual state of fear, but once we embrace the unconscious actions of many around us, the process of forgiveness becomes quicker and easier and we can once again enter a state of holding loving connections for others.

15- The Beautiful Bell

Finite and Infinite, seen and Unseen, nature and Consciousness are all aspects of our everyday existence whether we want to believe it or not. Physiologically, our bodies are the most complex living things on the planet, being morphed from the blueprint of our DNA and the raw materials of the earth every second of our living life. On top of this miracle, we are flowing with the Infinite, the Unseen, with Consciousness in ways that we will never fully understand. In yoga, it is believed that the Unseen enters into us through our nadis. The nadis are a complex interconnected nerve-like infrastructure inside the body with nodes that act like accumulating centers for the Unseen. Our nodes vary in size, with the seven largest of these nodes, called *chakras*, aligning along the spine starting from its base at the sacrum and extending all that way up to the top of the spine[39]. They allow us to uniquely parse the Infinite into smaller, more finite pieces that are needed to help us navigate the world around us. These pieces turn into our characteristics like survival, creativity, power, love, communication, intuition, and wisdom. In an ideal world, we allow the Infinite to flow through us unfettered, unblemished, which is achieved when our mind surrenders to the Infinite, but that state is difficult for

---

[39] See Table 1: Chakra Overview

87

even a holy person to hold indefinitely. Like a bell when struck sounds alive and beautiful, we, too, have the capacity to exist beautifully. We just need to realize that our physical tension, mental confusion, and emotional pain dampen our journey toward Holiness, and then work to refine it so that every step we take in life exists for the Glory of God.

16- More Will, Less Perfection

When we have even the slightest forward progression spiritually, God smiles upon us. The difference between forward progress and perfection is that when we progress forward, we are refining the opportunities in our life to make them better for ourselves and others. On the other hand, many times when we achieve perfection, it is at a cost, a cost to our health, our morals, and our servanthood. Our Soul guides us to continuously move forward, but our nature is geared to fit in, to win, to survive, to find perfection. The more dichotomy between the two, the more suffering in the mind. The Consciousness in the world today is rising, and as it does, the whisper of the Soul is more prevalent, causing confusion in the minds of many. Unless we find ways to surrender or let go of our nature, this confusion will only grow, as seen in the increasing rate of mental health conditions, which are even more prevalent in our younger adults and children. Since the rate of increase of Consciousness will only continue to grow, it is imperative that as yoga instructors, we help others find ways of releasing, surrendering, and letting go of their nature.

17- Lighting a Candle

Find time every day to become still, physically, mentally, and emotionally, because stillness leads us naturally into our Essence. When we find our Essence, we find patience, forgiveness, kindness, gentleness, peace, joy, and ultimately, love. The longer we are here, the deeper these spiritual threads weave into the fabric of our existence. The tighter our weave, the better example we are for the world around us. We don't have to say a word to anyone. We just need to be a shining example for others to see. Your stillness practice should be simple. Create a routine, a rhythm that tells your mind and body that it is time to be still, like lighting a candle and sitting for a few minutes. In this stillness, go inward as if you are falling into yourself, falling into your Essence, your Soul. This is less about you doing anything and more about letting it be done unto you. Feel your Inner Infinite expand into every cell of your body, every thought in your mind, and rest in the presence of your Self.

18- Find Your Inner Well

The world is ready for exceptional leaders who forge our way into the next phase of human evolution. This new world is a place of deep, loving connections between all people, creating a harmonious sea of humanity. In this world of coexistence, we see the importance of giving to receive, for when we love, we become "turned on" as Infinite instruments of God's Making. Every human has the capacity to serve in this way. They just have to look down into their spiritual well to find their sustaining source of life. At first, our well might feel very deep, because we are depending on our immature ego state to navigate the world around us, but with time, we find a mature ego state that bows to our Infinite within, causing our well to overflow. Find your inner Infinite source and share it!

19- Anatomy of a Spiritual Mind

The organ of the brain and, hence, the mind is the most complex living thing on this planet. Science has made amazing discoveries about its complexity, but there is still much to learn. When we process the world around us, we rarely appreciate all that is going on in the brain. If we break it down in an elemental way, there is the cerebellum at the lower back of the brain, the limbic system in the middle of the brain, and the neocortex, which is the curvy outer surface of the brain. When we look at the evolution of our brain, we started with a lizard brain consisting of the cerebellum and the spinal cord, allowing us to instinctively react to the world around us to stay alive. From here, we evolved into the mammal brain with the growth of the limbic system, our highly refined bells and whistles system, to help us process and regulate emotion and memory. More recently, the growth of the neocortex has propelled our advancement into higher cognitive functioning of thought and Consciousness. This anatomy is important if we are on a spiritual path, because it helps us understand the nuances of remaining fully conscious and loving, the complexities of a meditation practice, and that when we lose our mind, it's not even close to personal :-)! To simplify this even more, let's say we have three voices in our mind, the immature ego, the mature ego, and the Soul. The immature ego would come from the cerebellum, our reactive source, the mature ego from the neocortex, our Consciousness, and the whisper of the Soul from an arc that is created between the pineal and pituitary glands, our antenna into the Unseen, both situated at the top of the spinal cord with the pineal gland toward the back and the pituitary gland the front. Each of these aspects of our brain communicates with us at different intensities—the immature ego is a yell, the mature ego a chat, and the Soul a whisper. Therefore, when the immature ego is present, it is very hard to hear your Soul. Our charge is to find ways to recognize and manage the immature ego, so that our mature ego has a higher probability of serving the Soul.

20- The Human Body's Future

We are Infinite and finite at the same time on this Earth, for a short period of time compared to our Infinite existence, so celebrate the gift of your life every chance you get. Our whole life, we are called to find our Infinite, and when we do, we are a new Creation on this planet, because our mind sees with a new Collective Consciousness. Our immature ego sees this journey as going upward and yet our mature ego knows that it is a journey of falling, falling into our Infinite as our mature ego helps the immature ego to surrender. In today's state of evolution of the human body, this is still the path least traveled, the narrow path, which means that the mind is more driven by our primitive/reactive instincts than our Soul, our Consciousness. Each of our Souls have uniquely been identified to be here at this time of tremendous change, because deep within we have the fortitude, strength, and discipline to contribute to the evolution of the human body. If you are reading this, you are already on the path. All we need now is patience, the willingness to participate in God's Will as it naturally molds the future of man right in front of us.

21- Healthy Changes for the Body

If you want to live a long, healthy life, you will have to be kind and gentle to your body and mind. If we are not consciously working on this, our busy and overindulging society will cause us to place stresses on the body and mind that will pull us far away from our goals of health. We will have to be conscious of how our environment affects us and what healthy rhythms we need to sustain our health. To start the process, begin with evaluating and creating healthy rhythms for how you Breathe, Eat, Move, and Sleep, and then from here it only gets more complicated. For many, our environment is the tricky one, because it includes things out of our control, like our home life, work life, and social life. This is where our stresses generally begin, like stresses in our mind from our relationships and perceived responsibilities, or stresses in the body because healthy food is not readily available. To resolve these stresses, you will have to first become conscious of them, so become an observer of your environment and how it affects you, then make the appropriate changes to support healthy living.

22- From Satisfaction to Joy

Today our society has us longing for states of satisfaction, which are just temporary states of happiness. We pile these up during our day, hoping to find joy, but not even a million happinesses will add up to one ounce of joy. Our Soul calls us to joy, but our immature ego has us searching for satisfaction, satisfaction in our favorite drink or multiple drinks during the day, fast food or tasty treats, or even gossip about others, just to name a few. It is in our stillness that we realize our calling to find joy, because in our stillness, we find our Soul, and our Soul is guiding us toward a positive endpoint. When we have found our endpoint, we have found our purpose. Our purpose fills us with joy, and this joy leads us to love, and love is here to heal all of Creation.

23- Redecorating the Mind

Is it better to push or flow through life? It seems in today's world, we no longer see the benefit of flowing and almost even enjoy pushing ourselves through the day, because we can see the accomplishments getting checked off hour by hour, and these accomplishments satisfy our immature ego's demands. When we flow, we experience peace and are more aligned with the natural outpouring of God's Grace and Will, so why do we push more than we flow? We do this because our push is tied to our

93

immature ego, and the flow is tied to the Soul, and at this stage in our evolution, the mental presence of our immature ego far exceeds the presence of the Soul. It is the difference between a scream and a whisper. Therefore, the only way to hear the Soul is to reduce the scream or concentrate more on the whisper. Either way, it will take a commitment to change. The latter is an easier path for today, because all it takes is finding stillness and in your stillness finding a deep state of relaxation. From this state you can feel the presence of the Soul. The prior will take a lifetime of effort, because you are reshaping who you are today for a higher expression of yourself for tomorrow as you refine your immature ego into a mature ego. If you choose this path, you will need a teacher or a group of people to share your journey with to help validate your work and properly navigate the nuances of the journey ahead. If your house is your mind, it is like hiring an interior decorator and an architect to help you do some remodeling. Once you begin the process, you will need to periodically reflect on your progress, so that over time you realize the benefits of your efforts.

24- Finding Comfort in Discomfort

Our instinct is to survive, and we satisfy this instinct with comfort. Therefore, comfort is at the heart of our primitive existence. This instinct has been with us from the beginning as human beings, helping us define and maintain our identity, our "I," our primitive self. When we walk into a room, this is the side of us that asks, "Are we safe? Do we fit in? Are people judging me?, etcetera. Our next step as human beings is to move out of this primitive instinct mode to expand into a spiritual existence mode. To realize this, we will have to find comfort in our discomfort and accept that the journey ahead will take work to find and maintain our Self. From this newly evolved state, we will be in alignment with the Will of God and play an integral part in God's new Creation.

25- Healthy Rhythms

In order to see the magnitude of work that we are called into, know that our endpoint, as an instrument of God, will take a lifetime or more of effort. With this said, it is important to find patience with ourself and everyone around us along The Way. The key characteristics to our successful journey are discipline and rhythm, or many would just call this "finding a practice." The first step in the journey is to find a rhythm in your day for being still or contemplative. This is important, because for many the days are filled with business that keeps us from seeing the Glory of God in the world around us. The second is to find discipline in our rhythm. This discipline begins with hope, and with time hope leads to faith. It is our faith that guides us into the journey of our endpoint. This Knowing serves as our spiritual compass, steering our actions into alignment with the Will of God. When we venture off the path, our spiritual discontent grows to pull us back to the Truth, and when we are on the path as a reward or validation, we experience peace, joy, and love. Therefore, find healthy rhythms in your life and you will experience your highest form of existence.

26- Praying for Loved Ones

As contemplatives and mystics, we are called to find oneness with God, a feeling of falling into, through deep surrender, the essence of all of Creation. We begin with a practice that leads to an experience, and this experience is a feeling of complete integration with God. Initially, it is a feeling beyond our knowing, a newness that is so exhilarating that we desire to find it again, and again, and again. From this first initiation, by the Grace of God, we are awakened into a new body, a new mind. From this newness, our actions spring forth like water from a source of goodness, kindness, compassion, joy, and love, or like a lotus flower seed that has found its way out of the muck, through the water, and now rests on the surface, fully receiving the life-sustaining radiance of the sun. At this point, we have graduated out of a practice to become contemplatives or meditators. This is because we have already found our Way to the Creator. It is like a switch that we have found within us that we can turn off and on at any moment in time, while we sit to meditate or during our day. Our newness allows Creation to flow through us unfettered into the world around us, resulting in a beautiful prayer of healing for those that we love and touch during our day.

27- Finding Our Service

For most people, each day is a compilation of routines that benefit their social and work life. These benefits could include financial benefits to a company or reassurance to their ego of their social media presence. To change our routine from self-serving into service is to become conscious. A conscious being is someone always on the lookout for their purpose in the moment or over time, for they realize that life is about service and that loving service is our ultimate action. Our Consciousness comes from the Soul, and its intensity and truth are directly related to our ability to open our mind and heart to its presence. This softness can be found through moving from an immature to a mature ego state, where an immature ego always wants to take or to prove itself, and a mature ego always wants to give, to serve. The more we find our mature ego state, the more loving we are to ourselves and everyone around us. In this state we find resonance with all living things, meaning that 1 + 1 = 10 or that we have found communion with another. To be in communion with another is our highest state of service, because it always allows us to perfectly align with God's Will. We find ourselves here because we are open to our Soul, finding comfort in the Unseen and its infinite potential in this world.

28- Honing Your Intuitive Nature

Evolution is moving us out of the self and into the collection so that we can truly see the non-dual world that we live in, where One is all and all are One. To be intuitive means to know without words, to feel another. The connection starts in the organ of the brain, the mind, and ends in the heart, so at first we see and then we feel. We must not confuse this type of feeling with the ones we get from our primitive limbic system. No, this feeling comes from the Unseen realm, the Soul. We have many of these little experiences throughout our life, and maybe just think, "Why am I thinking that?" This is our introduction into the Unseen, into the Collective. As we deepen our love for all things, we will be called to hold the love for others, intuitively, to show them the way to love. By Universal Law, this is done unto us as our capacity to love grows. When we move from this introduction phase of our intuitive nature, it can be a bit disorienting. Many have documented this experience as an awakening, the Dark Night of the Soul, or a new profound Knowing, but once you graduate into this phase, you will never go back and will be called to hone your new intuitive faculty for the rest of your known life. This is the importance of a daily practice, so that we can find clarity and stability in our new world.

29- New Explorers

To have a true meditation practice, you have to be a brave explorer, not dissimilar to an ocean explorer standing on the dock getting ready to sail with his boat and crew. As captain, you must gaze out into the vastness of the deep ocean and mentally prepare for the journey ahead. You have to be willing to fully accept that there will be good days and challenging ones. At some level, deep down, you are driven by the newness that this experience will give to your heart and mind, and that your efforts will plot a course for many more brave explorers to follow. All true meditators know that Bravery is at the heart of a successful practice, for in the absence of bravery we will always find fear, and fear will always pull us far from our full potential as spiritual beings. The spirit is looking for a place to flow. To turn on this flow within us, we have to become a path of least resistance for the Spirit. To begin the flow, take on bravery. With bravery we become believers. All true believers love, and love will open the door to the Spirit.

30- Falling into the Depths of Communion

The organ of the brain is designed to help us operate our very complex body, safely navigate the seen world, and potentially integrate into the unseen realm. To understand its basic development, it turns on at week six as an infant and is fully developed by age twenty-five. To understand its basic function of thought, each thought rides on a highway of synaptic connections. There are about a quadrillion (1,000,000,000,000,000) synapses, and each synapse has about a thousand transistors in it—and it only gets more complicated from here. Yes, science has just scratched the surface of the brain. Now back to how we can best utilize our brain. Our first instinct is survival. Our mind will remain grounded in this immature ego state to help us navigate the seen realm until it feels safe. When it feels safe, the mind will begin to perceive the subtleties of the realm of Consciousness. The depths of this journey are dependent on the Grace of God, our environment, management of life experiences (maturity of ego), discipline, and life practices. The more we practice, the easier it is to venture into the depths of the Unseen and into the complex web of universal interconnectedness. The more mature the ego, the more willingness to refine our own pain and suffering. When we are able to hold this state of perfect existence, then by Universal Law we will be called to refine the pain and suffering of others. (If you are a mother, you already understand aspects of this Rule of the Universe.) We remain in this state of function until such a time that we are unable to hold the pain and suffering of others and then fall back into personal refinement mode. When we become stable, we will be called into Communion again and again and again. This is the highest function of a Conscious brain and the true journey of a Holy Person.

31- Being Fearless Explorers

Our life is a collection of individual journeys that take us from where we are now to where we plan to go. Over our lifetime, these journeys take on many different forms. They could include playing with friends, attending church, attending a birthday party, going to class, going to work, becoming engaged, getting married, having kids, picking up kids, taking vacations, walking the dog, and so on. The first time we experience each of these little journeys, we are more like explorers, because the journey is unfamiliar to us and there is an excitement in doing something new. Our charge in life is to never lose our exploring nature, even after we have completed the same journey one hundred times. To do this we have to move deeper into the present to see the inner workings in every moment in life. Maybe along our journey to walk the dog we notice the sky, the trees, the wind, and the sun more intensely and even feel more intimate with Mother Nature. When we are able to explore life in this way, it makes us feel alive. When we feel alive, we feel purposeful. When we have purpose, we feel content. Contentment leads to peace, and peace leads to joy and love. When we can hold joy and love for a period of time, we have become fearless explorers, and in this state we are limitless. May our inner explorer lead the way in all that we do today!

32- Seeing Your Infinite

We are more Infinite than finite, more expansive than limited, more whole than incomplete, so let us rejoice and be glad, for today is our day to see the truth! We start our life journey grounded in the finite world around us. This view is mostly based on our brain's interpretation of our senses. For most of our life, we are working to understand and fit into this perceived world. We start our journey recognizing the social component of our family, friends, school, work, or faith. Our priority is to synthesize this information so that our next step in the world appropriately aligns with the social norm. This process is molded deep within our DNA to help us survive and is our rhythm in life until we feel safe. Once we do, we begin a journey of contemplation, a conscious journey allowing us to fall into ourselves, into our Soul, into our Infinite. In this stage, we move out of the perceived duality of life and into wholeness, oneness, helping us to begin to see the non-dual world around us, the world of complete interconnectedness, infinite potential, and infinite possibilities.

33- Removing the Stain

When we release, we receive, because in a surrendered state, we become the perfect instrument of God's making. When we are tense, stressed, or in pain, we stop the flow of God's grace (Holy Spirit, prana, chi, kundalini, etc.), damping our full potential. This is why it is so important to practice surrender (i.e., Yoga Nidra), so we can witness and temporarily remove our blockages. With time, the practice leads to an Awakening, a Knowing that is profound and life-changing. With our first awakening, we see for the first time what it takes to remove a layer of mental illusion, and in that instant, we see clearer as we remove the stain that was once there. Over time, as our practice deepens, we become more efficient at removing the stains, bringing us closer and closer to The Truth with each practice.

34- Running with the Infinite

It's not that the Infinite isn't already flowing 100 percent through us at all times; it's that we are still learning how to sense and utilize It. Yes, we can get glimpses of the Infinite in our mind; we are just still learning how to hold it for more than an instant. The secret to holding it is Faith. When we have Faith that we are an Infinite being, we will receive the Infinite at all levels. Stop doubting your potential and you will realize that all things are possible.

Doubt stems from fear, and fear is at the heart of our primitive being, wired in at the core of our essence as a human being. Consciously or unconsciously, we are all evolving into an Infinite being but at a very gradual rate. For those of us with a passion to reach our highest potential in our lifetime, know that it's okay to stumble a bit, not dissimilar to how a child learns to walk—one step at a time. The Creator always celebrates when we try to receive the Infinite, the same way parents support their child as they learn to walk. With time we will find ourselves running with the Infinite.

35- The Power of Relationships

We are called to love and serve one another, for when we are with another out of love, God is able to Create in the world in infinite measure. We were not designed to walk this world alone. Our relationships with others help bridge a deeper connection with our inner voice and wisdom, helping us to find our way when we are lost. A mature ego realizes that there will always be work to do in aligning the Soul with the mind. This patient, forgiving mind embraces the challenges of our loving relationships as a way to navigate our actions back onto the well-lit path of God's Creation. In the absence of this realization, we might find the stubbornness of an immature ego mind holding us tightly on an incorrect course regardless of the consequences. Allow your loving relationships to move you from a tightly held bud with no eyes to see the world around us into an open blossom rejoicing to have found the Sun, the Creator, and the infinite path that is ready to be seen.

36- Invoke Your Inner Intelligence

Remove your inner resistance and let your Infinite intelligence flow. Our potential is endless, because deep within us is an Infinite intelligence, ready at all times to go to work in this Earthly Plain once we remove our resistance to its flow. This resistance is in the form of physical and mental dis-ease. Our physical resistance can be in the form of physical ailments or an overworking sympathetic nervous system, and is the easiest to control. If we are active, physical ailments occur from time to time and must be resolved as quickly as possible with body and energy work. Our environment, consisting of who we integrate with, what we watch, and what we listen to, directly impacts our nervous system. Environments that cause our sympathetic nervous system (fight, flight, or freeze) to remain on guard or to repeatedly fire create the greatest barrier to our Infinite potential. Our mental resistance is very complicated, and if we are a conscious being, it is something that we will work on for the rest of our life. It begins by finding your childlike mind again, a playful, simple mind filled with peace, joy, and love. Overlay on this purpose, and you have achieved a mature ego state. This is the doorway to surrender, and surrender is the doorway to the Infinite. In the absence of this, we will always fall into an immature ego state, a state filled with fear, doubt, control, and individualism. Once we find a mature ego state, we can begin the work of refinement.

Refinement of our own inner dis-ease (little and big traumas) and the dis-ease from those around us. This is the journey of a conscious being, a wise being, a mystic, a yogi or a yogini, and is the ultimate example of pure love.

37- Letting It Be Done Unto You

The Soul's goal is to help us "turn on" so that our actions better align with all of Creation. This is achieved when there is balance between the body, mind, and Soul. We begin the journey of balance when the body is removed of all its dis-ease and discomfort and the quality of the mind maintains a mature ego state. When this occurs, the Soul can begin its work of moving from the Unseen into the seen realm. If our body and mind were a guitar fully constructed and ready to be played, then our Soul would be the musician. When we are not in balance, the strings are out of tune, and our mind places a hand on the strings so that even if the Soul tries to play the guitar, it sounds muted and out of tune. With time we learn the importance of a healthy environment, healthy foods, and a healthy body. We respect the power of our primitive instincts, the effects of trauma, and how to maintain a relaxed state amidst troubled thoughts, and we realize our life purpose. When this occurs, we are balanced and aligned with the workings of the Soul, allowing us, as an instrument of God, to be played unfettered, at full capacity, spreading joy and love all over the world!

38- Living on Manna

Physiologically, the cells of our body take on food, water, and air to sustain our life. This is part of our gross nature for survival, but this only explains the seen realm. How does our body and the cells of our body integrate into the Unseen realm? Let's start with the fact that it is impossible for our finite brain to truly understand our Infinite Maker, but let's give it a go. With a consistent, highly refined practice of meditation, you will realize the edges of our Infinite Maker and how She is all encompassing in us and in everything around us. The formula for integration of the Unseen works like this: the more you release and surrender, the more you receive. To begin to help the finite brain understand this Unseen food, some have called it Manna, and it flows in the absence of our control. This Divine food provides infinitely more life-sustaining nourishment than our gross food, so if we are able to receive it for even an instant each day, we will realize perfect health in our physical body and mind, and from this a deep connection with our Soul.

39- Gross to Gentle

Our Consciousness is settle and our instincts are gross. Our basic instincts for survival start out as a binary reaction, if this, then that. A bunch of 0s and 1s, offs and ons. This design is needed for survival when running from a tiger or sensing if we are going to be ousted from the village, because there isn't much time to think or to be conscious when an actual life-threatening event is about to occur. Neither of these scenarios are very prevalent today, so in the absence of real threats, our gross nature will continue to scan our surroundings for similar threats, like family dysfunction, peer judgment, financial strain, and mental bullying or abuse. This is where the work begins. We are called to be settle, conscious, and objective with our reactions to life's events, because from this vantage point, we operate more from the inner whisper and less from our deeply integrated binary switches. Initially this might seem impossible, but with practice we begin to soften the edges of our reactive nature and awaken our contemplative nature to align our actions with God's Creation in every moment.

40- The Way, the Truth, and the Life

There is a WAY to get to the Father, and it is through attuning our body, mind, and Soul into its highest state of integration, where the three become one. The mind will have the greatest opportunity for refinement in most people's lives, so this should be a point of focus for many of us. The first step is to move through fear. To do this, one will have to realize that we don't get rid of it; we just deflate its importance or perceived potency and then have faith in the natural unfolding of God's Vision and our role in Her Creation. It's actually simple; we just need to believe in it. The second is to tame our primitive behavior, so that our actions are additive, like to move lust into love, and love into Creation. After graduating from these first two steps, one will be anointed with the power of Creation. At this point there is a fork in the road. One leads to individual power and the other to the collective power for all. The latter is the road less traveled but the correct turn for participation in Creation. Once on this path, by the Grace of God, we experience our metanoia and see the Truth. It's like cleaning off our glass lenses so things can appear sharper, crisper. Once we find the Truth, we can never go back. We find comfort in being a servant for Creation, because we have discovered how to hold God's Infinite love for ourself and all things around us. When we repeat this day after day, it will become our Life. This is our true purpose for living!

41- Going Beyond Your Mental Limits

If we want to get to the top of the mountain, we have to prepare the body physically and mentally and then have faith in the Soul to get us there. Our physical preparation is the easiest of the three. It will take planning, healthy eating, discipline, and patience in the repetitive action of feeding and toning the physical body for the journey. When we move into the next two stages, things get a bit complicated. The mental part of the journey depends on surrender, forgiveness, concentration, establishing a mature ego (finding your purpose), peace, joy, and love. The first stage is self-love, and once we master this, we will be called (initiated, awakened) into The Collection of Love (communion, love for all). To love yourself is to turn on God's instrument. Once the instrument is turned on, Consciousness will play the instrument in accord with the needs of Creation. The third and final stage is the hardest. It will require faith, our ability to hold our deepest surrender, so that our Soul can project into us the needs of Creation. If the mind is tone and mature, one will find bliss in participating in Creation, and if the mind is immature, the journey will appear to be infinitely difficult or impossible.

42- Moving into the Collection

Our first Knowing in this world is the knowing of the connection between the body and the mind. When we are able to tame or mature this little self, we are awakened into the collection of The All. This awakening is the realization of the Soul, the Big Self, and the role the three play together as instruments of God's making. The deeper the surrender of the little self, the purer the actions of the Big Self, where actions are our service and service is our purpose. There are two types of actions, those that align with Creation and those that don't. Every action has a repeating action or reaction, like ripples in the water from a rock. The action of the rock going through the water continues to impact the surface of the water even after the rock is not seen.

The Iroquois Indians believed that our actions today impact the next seven generations of people. If the action is fruitful, it will sustain itself into the future, and if it doesn't align with the Will of God, it dissipates over time. Be still a little bit every day to integrate your body, mind, and Soul, and from here listen for your inner whisper guiding your actions today toward the Will of God, and you will ultimately serve the collection of people around you.

43- Find Your Resonance

Our first stage in meditation is to find a deep surrender. When we surrender, we are able to soften the physical body and from this find a mature ego mind that allows the gentle nature of our Soul to integrate into our physical existence. In this first stage we are preparing ourselves, the instrument of God's design, for optimal participation in this world. This would be like if we were a bell and God had a hold of our handle in preparation for ringing us and our immature ego had a hand on the bell part, so that when God rings us, our full beauty as a bell would not be realized. Therefore, we have to move through surrender in order to participate in God's Creation. The second stage in meditation is to find our natural resonance, the frequency at which $1 + 1 = 10$ or higher, maybe even infinite. When we attune to our natural resonance, we are "turned on," and in this moment we are fully physical, fully spiritual, and at our highest potential. The third stage is beyond this world and is only realized by the Grace of God. We practice meditation because we know that it is not easy, that it is challenging, but that our practice leads us into refinement, and refinement into participation. It is our way of saying, "Thank You," to our Maker. Don't miss your meditation today :-)!

44- Spiritual Recalibration

The Holiest of human beings on this earth walk from where they are, call it their point A, to the Will of God, call it point B, in a straight line, rarely stumbling or straying from their path. For many, the journey to God can be a bit clumsy and uncoordinated. This diversion from God's chosen path for us comes from our immature ego focusing on itself over serving others. If the line between A and B is a rubber band in a relaxed state then the journey to B is effortless. If our immature ego pulls on the rubber band in one direction or the other and we divert from God's chosen path for us then tension and even distance will be added onto our journey to God's point B. This tension can be perceived as pain, suffering, or divine discontent and is our cue that we have left the chosen path and to realign our travels. When we react timely to these cues their reaction on our life is minimized, but when we get too far off the path and tension starts to build, the reaction back to our chosen path can be so great that it pulls us through the chosen path to the other side, where we are once again back in tension. Be still daily and your Chosen Path in life will be illuminated.

45- The Journey and the Pause

Our life starts at "A" and goes to "B." It sounds straight but actually meanders to and fro throughout our life. To see our progress, occasionally we need to pause and reflect, to be conscious. It's like when we are swimming head down in a lake: occasionally we have to look up to make sure we are moving in the right direction. Our Soul always knows The Way, but our instincts can direct us away from our ideal endpoint at any time. This is why finding our Consciousness, a little bit every day, lights the path toward our purpose and our actions for the day. To reinforce that we are heading in the right direction, our Soul will help us feel peace, joy, and love. When our movement is random, because our instincts are in control and we are moving away from our purpose, we will feel divine discontent. This is a powerful safeguard of communication between our Soul and our self (ego) to let us know that there is a more favorable direction to go. Find your pause every day so you can look up and clearly see your path to Consciousness.

46- Men, Holding the Foundation of Evolutionary Change

To realize our place within evolution, one must understand the complexities of achieving this next phase of human existence. It begins by understanding our individual journey and at the same time its complete integration with all things living. When the Flesh surrenders to the Soul, we begin to see and even feel our full potential as an instrument of Creation. In this moment there is a Knowing that we are completely insignificant (immature ego surrender) and fully significant (realization of a mature ego/purpose). To evolve is to refine—to take what is crude/raw today and make it better, more useful, more purposeful for tomorrow. Our finite mind sees what is crude as pain and suffering. To move beyond this we must turn on our refinery to process the pain individually, converting it into beauty, into love. In this exact moment, through our communion with all living things, each Soul in this universe sees our process of refinement and is able to utilize it within the evolution of their finite body. When we refine even a little bit every day, we are walking a fully conscious life, a loving life! This refinement is infinitely complex, but to try to capture it for the finite mind, yoga has given us the chakras, vortices where the Unseen enters into the seen through our human body. (He is fully Divine and fully Human; "I and the Father are one"[40]).

Conscious men and women work daily to refine their chakras, so that their Unseen can enter into this physical universe unfettered and unstained to maximize Its loving potential in the seen realm. If there are seven chakras, women have taken the upper four and men the lower three for their home base of work and refinement. The upper four are love, communion, intuition, and wisdom, and the lower three are survival, sex, and power.

At a forty thousand–foot level, it is easy to see that there is work to do. Women play the highest role in refining love in the Universe and even realize an intensity for refinement after their first child. Men are designed for battle and therefore are grounded in the chakras that need the most refinement, the first three. I pray that all fathers on this Father's Day are able to recognize the deep need for refinement of our animal instincts and their

[40] John 10:30

responsibility for carrying humanity into its next phase of evolution.

47- Awakening of Consciousness

On a beautiful starry night, our minds are intrigued by gazing out into the infinite. For generations, the mind has been fascinated with exploring the land, the sea, the sky, and space. This intrigue also finds us exploring the Unseen, the Infinite within, which has been driven from the birth of Consciousness around ten thousand years ago (Adam & Eve story) followed by an explosion of Consciousness in human beings over two thousand years ago across the planet. Since each human being sees through their unique lens of the world, it was their perspective of the environment (society, culture, physical location, friends, and family) at the time of the Awakening of their Consciousness that began the process of putting the pieces of Consciousness (seen and Unseen) back together that resulted in the over four thousand religions that exist in the world today.

48- Flowing into Diversity

God's Infinite Creation is full of contrasts. These contrasts help to prepare us for our journey into the depths of opposites. When we are able to hold opposites, we are ready to serve others unconditionally. To serve unconditionally is to love, and this level of service is where God is leading all conscious beings.

To begin the journey, we have to embrace the abundance of diversity that God has built into every aspect of Her Creation. We see diversity in the weather, plants (391 thousand), ethnic groups (650), cultures (3.8 thousand), animals (8.7 million), and microorganisms (1 billion). It is in everything around us and changing second to second. No, life is not static; it is fluid, flowing, and dynamic. When we are naturally flowing with the fluidity of our changing world, we are operating from a mature ego. Within this state, life will feel more like a dance with endless variations. To fall into this state of mind, we will need to be okay with losing control, the control of our perceived or favored outcome.

Our immature ego loves to feel in control or that it has the power to control life's outcomes, and it does this through our emotions. If our emotions are not able to drive the immediate desired outcome in the world around us, the immature ego will work to control even our own body and mind just for the pleasure of perceived control, but at the cost of holding tension and stress in the body, which over time can lead to chronic physical and mental disease. When we look at this characteristic consciously, it appears very dysfunctional, but we have to remember that this powerful survival instinct was designed as a short-term response to get us out of immediate danger and was never intended to be used long term or in the chronic state that we find used by many today. This powerful faculty of the brain was ingrained deep within based on the two million years of evolutionary experience for animal survival.

To move beyond this, we have to be less in our head and more in the moment. When we are truly present with the world around us, it is clear that our circumstances are not life or death today. This is why the media, which I no longer watch, enjoys tickling our minds daily with the worst possible scenario in the world around us and not the highest level of love or joy in the world around us. Our journey begins when we accept the changing world around us and fall out of survival mode to rest in the next phase of our evolution as conscious beings willing to serve others unconditionally.

49- Serving the One You Love

Once we realize that life is about serving one another, we will begin to fully experience the depths of peace, joy, and love in our life. Serving takes on many forms. First there is the general act of serving yourself, so that you can be the best version of yourself in serving others. Second, there is the quality of serving. This is dependent on the intention behind the act of serving. Are we serving from our mind, because we want others to think of us more highly for doing so, or are we serving from our heart, because at some level it is known that it helps us and the collection of all people? When we give from the heart, we give unconditionally to another, not expecting anything in return. This is the ultimate expression of serving. When we enter into a relationship with another, at first there is the physical connection, but with time there develops an Unseen connection, a superhighway of sharing all that is known and Unknown with the other. This is what is meant by being in communion with another, because we are able to complement the needs of our significant other, and this is love!

50- The Amplitudes of the Mind

Our brain is the most complex organ in our body and continues to evolve over time, helping us to perceive the seen and Unseen universe around us. For many, the journey of the mind is grounded in the seen with occasional glimpses into the Unseen. When we are ready to move deeper into the Unseen, it is imperative that we fully understand how the brain operates, what its limitations are, and how to maintain its optimal state of health, in order to minimize unnecessary behavioral health issues. When we journey from the seen into the Unseen, we are moving from the finite into the Infinite. Since our brain is finite, to see the Infinite, we need to be conscious.

After years of practice and by the grace of God, one day we will find ourself standing at the doorway of the Infinite looking in (Savikalpa Samadhi). How do we get through this doorway? Imagine the mind as a rectangular wall, and on its surface are all of our thoughts, memories, and sensory feelings, each extending from the wall's surface with their own amplitudes dynamically changing second to second depending on our mental focus and external sensory exposure. This faculty of the brain allows us to perceive and integrate into the seen realm. If everything perceived in the seen realm extends off of the wall, then

117

the doorway into the infinite is within the height of the paint extending from the wall. This tiny amplitude of higher Consciousness is at the foundation of every thought the brain can have. When you find the faculty to rest in this sliver of Consciousness, you will begin the journey into the vastness of all of creation, seen and Unseen. If you are able to find a quiet mind that is a gift. For many, it will be easier to find a part of the brain to hang out in, a safe place that comprises a collection of all of your peace, joy, and love experiences, allowing you to experience physical, mental, and emotional relaxation longer than just a few minutes. This is true for those that are still working through Big T traumas. With the help of neuroscience, we now have a better understanding of where our thoughts in the brain reside, which is called our *brain map*.

51- From Individual to Communion

Through a force of higher Consciousness, we are called to collectively participate with one another, to be in communion with all things created. Our effectiveness in holding this highest state of communion with others is realized only after we master our inner self, the ego. This mastery is a journey of moving our ego from an immature to a mature state. Our immature state sees life as a competition with winners and losers, us and them. We find ourselves using "I" and "Me" way too often, versus realizing that every conscious experience by all living things in this universe is experienced by all and held by all.

52- Mastery of Body & Mind Leads to Mastery of Mind & Soul

Connecting the seen with the Unseen is our overall purpose in life. Since we perceive the seen through our mind, and our Soul is the aspect of ourselves in the Unseen, we will need to master how to use the mind to see into the Unseen. When we see with these New Eyes, our purpose becomes clear, allowing our actions to flow with all of Creation. To achieve this level of mastery, we will need to establish a daily practice. This practice begins with mastery of the body and mind and leads us into mastery of the mind and Soul. Our practice of body and mind helps us to realize the external stresses that arise from our culture, the people we associate with, environmental toxins, the food we eat, not moving the body, or improper sleeping. These stresses get stored in the body physiologically and mentally, like when we find ourselves holding tension in our neck and shoulders.

A daily practice of movement that allows the mind to concentrate on our dis-ease or discomfort in the body and then using the breath with gentle pulsating movement or static holds to facilitate removing the dis-ease is a beautiful gesture of our willingness to someday fully participate in Creation. From our daily practice, the mind will learn how to concentrate on a physical goal and watch it manifest in the physical world and at the same time show us how to direct our desires to form positive change in the body. Both of these experiences help refine and stabilize the mind for our next level of mastery.

When we graduate through mastery of the body and mind, by the Grace of God, we will be called to journey into the mastery of the mind and Soul. In this practice we tune the mind to see through our external stresses in life to witness the subtle vibrations of the Unseen, not dissimilar to how a microscope works. You will know you are on this path because you will sense a level of Divine Discontent, a Knowing deep within that there is more, more to learn, more to do, and more to life.

53- Finding and Holding Your Conscious Mind

A non-conscious mind's first instinctive reaction is always to survive. This is wired deep within our DNA and at the core of every living animal. This pre-wiring helps us to react as best as possible to stressful situations to stay alive. We know we are in survival mode when we are fear filled. Fear always causes us to fall into the pre-wired survival state. If you have ever said, "Why do I keep doing this?" or, "Why can't I stop this habit?", it is because you are in survival mode. Our society today, like our media, movies, and even our religion, love to hold us in states of fear, because from this state, we are predictable and malleable. In a full fear response, our IQ drops in half. Therefore our mind is more apt to listen to what someone else is telling us to do versus coming up with a conscious solution on our own. Our journey toward full Consciousness is a life-long practice. Our practice should move us out of tension and into relaxation, physically, mentally, and emotionally. When we are able to hold this state for even a couple of minutes, the mind perceives the absence of fear and when fear is removed we will be graced with experiencing Consciousness—Consciousness of Self (Soul) and Consciousness of the Whole (Communion). This is the beginning of a non-dual mind, a mystical mind.

54- Mastery of Intimacy

In order to hold Consciousness, we have to master intimacy. Mastery of intimacy is the culmination of years of practice of holding the love of another, our deepest Knowing for being in communion with another. For many it started with the unconditional love of their mother or family member, and from here we mirrored this example in our relationships with others—our friends, our significant other, or the one we marry. After years of practice falling in and out of this highest vibration that a human being can hold for another, we refine our skills to hold this intimacy with our Creator. For it is through this connection that we reform who we are as human beings, accelerating our evolution into the highest form of Consciousness and purpose on the planet.

55- Having Faith in Creation

In order to allow God to flow through us unfettered, we will have to realize that all that happens to us during our lifetime is not personal, not personal at all. The actions of the world and others around us are just a part of Creation, the overall intelligence of the Universe. Yes, Creation is metamorphosing from one instant in time to the next, based on the collective Consciousness of the Universe in this moment in time to create the next moment in time. To take things personally is to control, and to control is to go against Creation. This doesn't feel right because it goes against our most powerful instinct: survival! God is calling us to move way beyond this state of mind and into a state of Consciousness. When we rest in states of Consciousness, we have Faith in Creation and rise above our fear to flow unfettered into the next moment in time.

56- Feeling the Flow of God

At some level we are all called to witness the Awesomeness of the Creator. In that moment, the Almighty will be inescapable, omnipresent, and flowing! This is because the Creator is in us, around us, and flowing through us at all times. This is possible because She is in the seen and Unseen of all things in this universe and beyond. When a person's flow is high their surrender is high. To maximize The Flow, we will need to remove tension in the body and stabilize our mind and emotions. This is yoga. This is truly what it means to surrender. We are not the creators of this world, but our actions, in participation with The Will of God, are designed to play a part in Creation. Learn your full potential for what it means to be an instrument of God and practice turning on your participation so you can witness the Pure Flow of God in and around you.

57- Moments of Pure Glory

What a blessing to have the life of Jesus as a model for our own life. This is a monumental example of how to devote your life to God and, from this devotion, reform the face of the Earth. His daily service of peace, joy, and love for others became an example for all to see. This purest form of service can only be realized in the absence of an immature ego, the deepest level of humility, or, as the Bible says many times, your deepest level of surrender. This perfect state of existence brings us closer to God so that our actions become unfettered and our purpose pure.

To find and maintain this state of surrender, you will need a practice to show you "The Way"! Your practice should show you how to surrender physically, mentally, and emotionally. This is why I fell in love with the science of yoga, because it shows us the path, the nuances, and the glory! Let me be clear: this journey will take many lifetimes, but once we are on the path we will begin to see with New Eyes the awesomeness of our non-dual universe and become Initiated, Awakened, and Confirmed into God's purpose for us. The further we travel the more challenging the road ahead becomes. You will see the highest peaks and the lowest valleys, but if you can maintain your state of surrender along The Way, you will be rewarded with moments of pure Glory.

58- Finding Yourself Within Yourself

When we are looking for something, we may never find it, but if we surrender to the possibility of finding it without looking, it will always be revealed. The difference is the level of the ego present in the search. An immature ego constantly believes that it is in charge of our next moment in life, so in the absence of this ego, we realize more of the Soul, and from this viewpoint we clearly see that what we were looking for has already been found.

59- Finding Calm Amid the Storm

Experiencing a calm mind is easier than we imagine, even if our life is extremely busy and full of more to-dos than we have time to do. Yes, our calm mind is with us at any moment. We just need a longing for it. After your mind desires calm and can hold this state for even ten seconds, you will find yourself in the moment, present in time and place.

To move deeper into this calm mind, slowly begin to lengthen your exhale as you maintain the length of your inhale. Maybe your inhale is four seconds, and your exhale is eight seconds. Do this for sixty seconds, and then let the breath come back to normal and just be present with your body and mind in this moment. Scan the quality of the body and mind, and see if you can release and relax just a bit more. Now be grateful that you are the most complex living thing on this planet, a gift to you in this life.

Cultivate self-compassion for all that you do in life, and know that what you do is exactly enough. Feel compassion for every living thing on this planet, and know that all things living in life struggle just like you do. Now feel connected to every living thing on this planet and in this universe and know that at some level, we are all one, super connected as God Creates the next moment in time and that, in some way, we are participating in this Creation. Find peace in your participation and begin to flow with the Spirit, releasing and letting go at an even deeper level. Feel light, open, and free. Feel like you are rising up into a bright cloud that is filled with peace, joy, and love, but mostly love. Now rest and just be.

60- Flowing Into God's Hand at Work

Figuring out how to flow in life is our ultimate purpose, for when we flow, we are participating in the Will of God. This sounds simple on the surface, but there is nothing simple about the workings of our mind with its layer upon layer of memories, sensory excitement, and thoughts. Therefore, to get to a state of flow, our mind must be able to attain and maintain states of calm and focus, because from this state, it is easier to witness the seen and Unseen workings of Our Maker. When we are able to realize God's Hand at Work, even for an instant, we are witnessing a slice of the Infinite. This witness will lead to the most intense intimate experience our human body can realize, and it is from this reward in the mind that we have the desire to find it again.

61- Seeing Through the Noise

When does the Soul enter the body? Is it preloaded by God at the point that two people fall in love? Is it tied to the physical act, or is the Soul less individual and much more collective, so that all life just falls into it at birth? If it is individual, does it take an outrageous amount of Unseen energy to create the physical bond? These questions are asking how the Unseen realm integrates into the seen realm.

We know that physically, when the body experiences an orgasm, over thirty parts of the brain are active.[41] Physiologically, both the sympathetic and parasympathetic nervous systems fire at the same time, and our happy hormones get released (oxytocin, dopamine) for pleasure and bonding to the mate. Is it a coincidence that the yoga teachings for experiencing Samadhi, the highest state of union of the body, mind, and Soul, are that the practitioner find balance in the sympathetic (pingala) and parasympathetic (ida) nervous systems, allowing Divine Energy to ascend up the spine (sushumna)? Probably not. The only difference is the release of hormones as a product of an orgasm. These hormones create so much mental noise and chatter that the massive presence of the Creator is muted or completely drowned out, and therefore not realized consciously. If this is the case, what a great design for a patient God to assure that one day Their Creation (mammals) would feel Their presence. With a personal

---

[41] (atlas bio med)

practice of contemplation/meditation (sadhana), we are able to heighten this realization through learning to soften and manage the noise in the mind, so that the presence of the Creator can be seen at all times.

62- Become the Masterpiece

When we master meditation, we experience our highest state of existence, peace, joy, and love. Our practice helps us to build this foundation deep within our existence. From this perspective, we are more conscious of how our natural instincts limit the existence of these states in our life. No, this limitation is not personal; it is just the part of us that we are still working to refine and remold. It is important that these steps of transformation be deliberate and purposeful and not harsh or critical. Yes, it is important that we are patient with our transformation and do not make it a race. We just need to define our course for life and purposefully walk it. Just like how a sculptor, over time, can take a square stone and work to transform it into a masterpiece, we too, with practice over time, will take who we are today to refine it into God's Masterpiece.

63- Happiness to Joy

When we see life through an unfettered lens into God Consciousness, we witness the true meaning of joy and live a joyful life. If we live life in the absence of this intimate connection with God or outside of our purpose, we only experience happiness. What is the difference between happiness and joy? Our happy experiences in life are generally short-lived experiences of pleasure and lack inner fulfillment and joy. This is why a thousand happy experiences will never add up to even one joy-filled experience. Happy experiences are created from our immature ego, and joy filled experiences are created from the Will of God. When we align with the Creator, our loving actions are multiplied, not added. One plus one does not equal two; it equals one thousand because of love. Therefore, the easiest way to find joy is through love and purpose. When we love ourselves, we find joy in ourselves, and when we love another, we find joy in life. What is the quickest way to love? You have to lose control, remove fear, and then have hope and Faith in God.

64- Finding Your Divine Resonance

God is connected to us, in us, whether we realize it or not. She brushes by the surface of our existence when we get a little tear in our eye from watching the sun rise, looking deep into the eyes of a baby, or watching birds fly across a vast sky. It is in these moments that there is a deep Knowing, a point in time when time stands still, allowing us to intimately connect with God Consciousness. This is one way that God softly says to us, "I am with you and in you." If we want to purposefully brush up against the surface of our Infinite Maker, we will need a meditation or contemplation practice, the deepest state of physical, mental, and emotional relaxation. This is what is meant by surrendering to God, for it is in these moments of contemplation that our special puzzle piece, our purpose, can more easily be seen. When we realize our purpose, our actions become additive to the Will of God, increasing the amplitude of God's ripple for the expansion of love in the universe. Finding our purpose is at the core of our existence, and when we are able to find it, we strike a divine resonance with God's Creation. The beauty in finding our path to complete integration of the body, mind, and Soul is that when we do, God shares our path to this highest state of existence with all other living things in Her Creation.

65- Your Seven-Story Building

If Consciousness comes from or is God, then we know when it began, at least 13.7 billion years ago when the universe was created. So the real question is, how does it integrate into the universe, into life, into us? Did it begin with single-celled life, around 3.7 billion years ago,[42] when birds and mammals developed larger brains, around 200 million years ago, or with *Homo sapiens*, around 200,000 years ago?[43] It begins when life is able to receive God Consciousness and then act in accordance with its Will. This sounds simple and yet is super complex. Yes, the evolution of our brain is moving us from reactionary (instincts/nature) to more conscious every day, and yet, most people are still grounded in their instincts.

---

[42] (Reber)
[43] Paul Thagard PhD, "When Did Consciousness Begin?" *Psychology Today*, January 11, 2019

One way to measure how conscious you are during your day is to study your actions. Start by thinking of your mind as a seven-story building. The first three floors are dedicated to our survival instincts, where the first floor is our instinct to fit in, many times driven by our material desires, the second our primal desire to recreate, and the third our desire to dominate and control. Then the top four floors are dedicated to our conscious actions, with the fourth being our passion to love, the fifth our passion to commune with others, the sixth our passion to recognize the workings of God, and the seventh our passion to integrate into God's non-dual universe. Now ask yourself, "What floor does my mind hang out on every day?" Don't worry if you believe that you are more grounded in the first three floors, because this is our unconscious homebase. It will take conscious work to get to floors four and higher. It's like you have a rubber band tied to you as you walk up the stairs of your seven-story mind. The higher you go, the harder it is to stay on that floor or state, but the more we practice going to the higher floors, the easier it becomes with time to stay there, so don't be afraid of working a little bit every day to fully realize your little part in life.

66- Turning Off the Autopilot

We have all heard the phrases, "die to self" and "surrender to self." If the self is your Soul, then what aspect of our existence is doing the dying or surrendering? If we use the word *refine* instead of *die,* does that make it easier to answer? If so, then what part of us do we need to refine? If at the end of the day these phrases were given to help us better align our actions with the Will of God, then what part of our mind controls our actions or even begins to recognize that our actions were supposed to align with something anyway? Is this our consciousness, the part of us that has a direct connection with our Soul and makes us different from animals? If we find out the opposite state of being conscious, do we have our answer? Is this what it means to be unconscious or unaware of your actions? Is this an autopilot state? Is this our instinct, our nature, and if so, who's doing the driving in these states? If the definition of *ego* is "the part of the mind that mediates between the conscious and the unconscious and is responsible for reality testing and a sense of personal identity," then it's not the ego. It's a part of us that has not matured into this state of the ego. Then the answer is that we need to refine the mind from an immature ego state to a mature state, a state that recognizes its purpose, so that its actions align with the Will of God.

67- Finding the Puzzle Piece

To surrender is to be turned on as an instrument of God. When we are turned on, we have realized the highest level of integration of the Body, Mind, and Soul. We are fully integrated and fully alive.

Why is it that we are at our best when we release and let go? It is because from here, we are able to see that we are but a speck of the total, a fraction of the whole, and that our work in this life is to fulfill the fraction and not the whole. Why is this often a challenge? It is because we exist mostly in our nature, the fear-based side of us that wants to control the outcomes in life and not flow with it.

The good news is that we are evolving out of our natural instincts and into Consciousness. With this Consciousness, God has gifted us views into the whole so that we can see our tiny part in it. Many times our enthusiasm for realizing aspects of the whole pulls us into participation with things outside of our purpose, and we lose sight of the special fraction that God has gifted us in this life. Surrendering always helps us to fall back into ourself, into the perfect puzzle piece that we were designed to be.

How do we know when our actions are aligning with our purpose? We will feel joy deep within. It is easy to determine when your actions do not align with the Will of God, because you will feel dissonance, frustration, and anger. This is usually when we are trying to control something that does not align with our purpose in life, our fraction of the whole. Find a way each day to fall into yourself, into your Soul, because from here your actions will always align with God and your unique puzzle piece.

68- Refining Your Existence

We are just a speck of Creation and yet fully integrated into the Creator. When our mind begins to see beyond the physical, it will naturally connect with the Unseen realm of the Creator through our Soul. This natural evolution is what we were called to be, physically separated yet fully one, and is the act of being in communion, a faculty of the mind that allows us to perceive beyond our instincts, our nature to connect deeply with our Soul. When we are conscious in this state, a doorway opens up into the Infinite of Creation, and we are able to see the connection of our oneness. This feeling brings us back into our heart center, our balance point of the human instrument, so we can realize what it means to be fully conscious and fully physical. With time and patience, we are able to hone this faculty of the mind to remain in deep concentration with no emotion, so that the mind can retain fragments of Total Consciousness, allowing our actions today to naturally flow with the Will of Creation.

For most, this journey is not designed to be walked alone. There will be many mentors, friends, and loved ones in our life that allow the journey to be realized, those who are there to hold our opposite long enough for us to refine this aspect in our life on our own. The work of self-refinement is important because when we don't hold our opposite, then we burden another Soul to hold it for us in the meantime. This Soul connection with another is like an ethereal string between two Souls and hence two beings, so if you want to do your mentors, friends, and loved ones a favor, find a way each day to refine yourself, the beautiful instrument of God's making. Explore your vastness! Refine your existence!

69- Supporting the Potter

A potter starts with a vision of their end product before they get started. Is their vision a vase, plate, or coffee mug? What type of clay body is the best to use, earthenware, stoneware, or porcelain? Yes there is much thought that will need to go into the design stage of this creation before the wheel starts to turn and the hands touch the clay. And yet, the design is only part of the whole. The body of the end product is directly related to the quality of clay used, because it affects the workability, firing temperature, and porosity of the completed product[44]. The higher the quality the easier it is for the potter to attain their vision. If the potter was your Soul and the clay your physical body are you eating the highest quality food today so that your Soul has the greatest potential to Create you in the image of God's Vision? Are you at the highest level of participation for your Maker? We are such an awesome gift, the most complex creature on this Earth, and have unlimited potential from where we are today to be the perfect form of God's Vision. Take time each day to be conscious of what you put into your body, so that you can attain your highest level of existence during our visit here on Earth. Laugh, love and celebrate for you are your own gift this Christmas Season.

---

[44] The Basics of Pottery Clay, Beth Peterson, 12/12/2019

70- Illuminate Your Path to Eternity

When we are still and have the will to fall deep into the hands of God in a state of surrender, we enable the instrument of God's making, our body, to see more clearly the immensity of all of Creation and our place in it. When we enter this state void of emotion, we have a better chance of understanding how dichotomies or opposites play their role in the universe. Why would our loving God Create good and evil when all we are called to be is good? Is the propensity with time for good and evil to get closer or further apart? Do we only realize the depths of love through also holding its opposite?

Jesus gave us so many lessons and examples of how to live life to its fullest through service to God the Almighty when he died on the cross for our sins. In complete communion with all of God's people, He held His love in one hand and our sins in the other, because his Body was prepared to hold the deepest of opposites on this earth. The ripples of His actions long ago have sparked the work of the Holy Spirit to continue to help us to hold these opposites while in communion with one another today.

To understand this, we must first recognize that good and evil are real. We definitely see it in the seen realm and can only begin to imagine its works in the Unseen realm. The safest way to traverse this terrain is through cultivating a highly refined mind, a mind that has the capacity to concentrate and meditate, where meditation means the ability to allow the Divine to flow through you unfettered.

135

So if you feel called to serve God and called to follow in the footsteps of Jesus or a Holy person, work daily to find the depths of God's love in your heart and mind and hold it, and you will illuminate a crystal clear path toward eternity for all to see.

> Speak, Lord, I'm listening.
> Plant your word down deep in me.
> Speak, Lord, I'm Listening,
> Please show me the way![45]

71- Stages Back to a Perfect Mind

Many will find their mind in a mature ego state for the first seven years of their life. During this time, the mind sees a non-dual world full of joy and love, and humans of this age want to celebrate life through playing, laughing, learning, and sleeping. These seven years are important because they form the foundation from which we build our relationship with God. The more developed the foundation, the easier it is for God's instrument to find God after they go through puberty (years seven through fourteen). During these years, our mind sees the duality (opposites) of life. As this duality builds (immature ego state) in the mind, we add layer upon layer of illusion, moving us further from the Truth and further from God. In this illusionary state, we will experience fear, and this fear will cause us to want to control. When we are unable to control, we will experience pain and suffering, and from

---

[45] "Speak, Lord, I'm Listening." Words and music by Gary Ault. Arranged and performed by Dave Rieves

here, the rabbit hole begins. Less perceived control drives more fear, and with more fear, more pain and suffering, and so on. When we find ourselves on this path, we need to remember God's training from the first seven years in life, for our inner child will always lead us back to God.

> The wolf shall dwell with the lamb, and the
> leopard shall lie down with the young goat, and the
> calf and the lion and the fattened calf together; and a
> little child shall lead them.
> —Isaiah 11:6

As we remove the illusion, we move ourselves back to a state of non-duality, oneness with all things. From this state, when we sit in stillness with God, we will hear Her gentle whisper again and see the peace, joy, and love that surrounds us. Find this perfect state of mind and find your oneness.

72- Holding Opposites

As our mind evolves, it generally moves from noticing ourself and caring for ourself to noticing others and caring for others. Since our origin is from the Unseen realm where all is one, one Spirit in communion with one another, caring and loving for others is our natural state of being. When we arrive here, we find abundant joy and love in the heart and peace in the mind. We find our dharma, our purpose in life. No, it's not to be a millionaire, or famous on TV. It's to be one with all things.

Our first step in participating in God's Creation is to transform our own pain and suffering into joy, love, and peace. Along this journey, we are moving from an immature ego state to a mature ego state. To accelerate our transformation, we might find ourselves drawn to nature, enjoying a sunrise, or enjoying time in stillness with ourselves. Our natural calling with time is to be one with all living things on this Earth and in the Universe (to be in communion). Why do we need to be one with other living things? This state is needed to accelerate the formation of God's Creation. When one learns how to transform their own pain and suffering, they are called to show others how to do the same.

Mothers get this state better than anyone, because of the natural state of communion they are in with their newborn. Yes, they literally get plugged into the people that they host in their bodies for nine months. When do we know we are ready? Once we are able to hold a mature ego, we are ready to hold the opposites of others. Take Jesus, for example, His ultimate love for us was to hold our pain and suffering, our sin, our opposites. Find a way to be that perfect image of God's Making, through working to remove tension and disease from your body, maintaining a stable mind, maturing the ego, and connecting deeply with your Soul. From here, you will find yourself participating in God's Creation.

73- Believe to Receive

Finding the balance between higher states of Consciousness and our nature is what we are called to hold today so that future generations of people may realize a deeper connection with God. When we hold these opposites together, we place demand on the organ of the brain to look deeper into the vibrations of the Universe and begin a process of deciphering that which is there, the Whisper of God all around us. It is from this state that we find a New Mind, a New Creation, a New Life.

To begin the journey, one will need a practice of refining the mind, meditating, or contemplating. We all know that the organ of the brain controls thought, emotion, memory, touch, motor skills, vision, breathing, temperature, hunger, and every process that regulates our body,[46] but where is the Whisper of God in all of this? How do we see, feel, and interact with God Consciousness? The first step is to learn how to reduce the noise of our nervous system, thoughts, emotions, and senses, the second step is to find God's Whisper, and the third step is to decode its meaning. All of this takes time, a lifetime, or lifetimes, but it is exactly what we are called to do. If this is what it means to meditate or contemplate, we can see that a daily practice is the minimum needed to begin the journey. It is a very complex process, and yet it is exactly

---

[46] Johns Hopkins Medicine, "Anatomy of the Brain," https://johnshopkinshealthcare.staywellsolutionsonline.com/Conditions/Neuroscience/About/85,P00773

what God has designed us to do. Yes, it is deep within us, and all we have to do is Believe to Receive!

74- God Speaks Within Us

For today, if we truly want to see God clearly, we should look through the heart, for the development of the brain is still evolving. When we take things personally (immature ego) or are filled with fear for the future (false control), we are like fledgling children learning to walk. Don't worry, this is all part of the process as we learn to tune the organ of the brain and hence the mind away from an immature to a mature ego state, because when we stay in an immature ego state, we keep our nature or primitive instincts on alert in survival mode.

Let's be honest: the only thing today that many have to worry about surviving is our own mind and its silly thoughts, so to tune it, we have to find our Consciousness within. Let's define Consciousness: it is "the inner sense of what is right or wrong in one's conduct or motives, impelling one toward right action: to follow the dictates of conscience."[47] This is a good start, but let's go one step further and define Consciousness as God Consciousness, the Presence, The Flow, The Dance of God within us. This would include the above definition and infinitely more. This presence of God is but a Whisper lightly flowing in all aspects of our being. When did we start to feel the presence of God within us? Our minds will

---

[47] "Conscience," Dictionary.com,
https://www.dictionary.com/browse/conscience

have to decide. Would it be: always, 13.7 billion years ago when the universe formed, when single-celled life began about 3.7 billion years ago, when animals such as birds and mammals developed larger brains around 200 million years ago, when *Homo sapiens* existed 200,000 years ago, or when the human culture became advanced around 3,000 years ago.[48] If you think that God created the universe for us, then it would be the latter example, and if you see God's creation to be infinite, then it would be more in line with the first one, "Always."

This means we are all spiritual beings trying to figure out what it means be human, more so than human beings trying to figure out what it means to be spiritual. Yes, our Soul has been around for a long time and God has blessed us all with an opportunity to realize 4 percent of Her Creation through our physical body. My prayer for all beings is that they walk a conscious path on this earth with their nature in a surrendered state and their Soul leading the way, so that they can clearly see and begin to participate in the beauty of God's infinite Creation. To find ourself, we must first lose ourself.[49]

75- Taming the Limbic System

After millions of years of hardwiring, our brains are experts on trust and distrust. When interacting with others, our brains sense whether we can trust the person

[48] Paul Thagard, PhD, "When Did Consciousness Begin?" *Psychology Today*, January 11, 2019
[49] Matthew 10:39

in front of us or not. If we can, we will open up, and if we can't, we will close down. If we sense trust, our prefrontal cortex (Ajna Chakra) is active along with the feel-good bio chemicals like dopamine, oxytocin, and endorphins, giving us a sense of well-being, enabling us to begin the journey of being in communion with another. In this state, the two are co-creators of the conversation, which opens their minds up with a multiplier greater than two, allowing them to have foresight and to see into the future.[50] On the other hand, if we sense distrust, we move to a different part of the brain, the amygdala (almond shaped, located in the limbic system, emotional processing center), which keeps us on guard so that we can appropriately determine the level of reaction needed to keep us safe. Yes, this is our sympathetic nervous system at work helping us to not think but to react to the situation, which is either to fight, flight, or freeze. In this state, the body will release cortisol, epinephrine, and norepinephrine designed to help us win the battle in the moment, but this is not a state where we want to remain in for very long. When we remain in environments (home, work, social, news) that are not trustworthy for extended periods of time, our distrust response fires repeatedly, and in this chronic state we reduce our telomere length, which shortens our lifespan. When we are unable to avoid these environments, a daily practice of meditation will tone the brain to help us remain in a state of well-being, extending our lifespan. It is critical that we become familiar with our

---

[50] Richard D. Glaser, PhD, "The Neuroscience of Conversations," *Psychology Today*, May 16, 2019

nature, so that we can evolve into our next state of existence.

76- Yoga Is Like a Flower

Learning the art of yoga is like how a flower grows from the ground up and then one day blossoms onto this Earth with radiance, delicateness, and poise. Its action to the world is that from a seed, it evolves into what it was designed to be by God, a radiance of color in the world, an example of intricate design, and an acceptance of grace. It surrenders to its environment, because it humbly sees that it is just a piece of a bigger picture. From our surrender, we see the path, walk the path, and then become the path for our Creator. It may seem that we are struggling as we transform through each stage of our existence from seed to stem, creation of leaves, and ultimately a bloom, but in the end, we are grateful for our journey of transformation, because we feel the love of being in communion with all of God's Creation.

77- Transforming Our Existence

When we surrender, we transform, and when we control, we transmit. God calls us to serve as instruments in Her Creation. She gave us many beautiful examples, and mine is Jesus. To surrender, we must flow into the changes around us, soften, and then just BE. In the absence of focusing on the work to establish this state, our instinct will always win over, which is to control, because in the past, being in control meant surviving.

So how do we learn to transform? It starts by finding more ways to flow with what is going on around us physically, or as I do, say, "Ignorance is bliss," and turn off the news :-). Reducing this noise in our mind is a big first step. The second step is to learn to transform our own pain by working with our body. This means having a yoga practice that refines the muscle-skeletal system to release (transform) any stored physical pain and suffering. After at least a year of this practice, you are ready for step 3: transforming the mind. This is like going from playing checkers to chess. It is complex. To transform your own pain and suffering in the mind, you will first need to master concentration (sutra 1.2).

> Yoga is the ability to direct the mind exclusively toward an object and sustain that focus in that direction without distractions.
> —Sutra 1.2

This is not the natural state of the mind, because our senses are wired directly into the brain and therefore comprise most of our mental processing. To master concentration, we have to become experts on how to turn down or off the senses in the mind temporarily. In yoga, this is called Pratyahara. Now, with a soft mind and the ability to direct it, we can begin the journey of opening up the mind to the flow of Divine Energy consciously. This is food for the brain from our Soul and has the ability to heal (transform) the scars in the brain and thus remove the pain and suffering associated with it. Step 4 is to learn to

144

be in communion with others, to hold ourselves in loving union with another. (By the way, this includes even those that we might think we hate today, sorry.) When we have mastered this, we will be ready servants to follow Jesus and transform the pain and suffering of others. Yeah, if you are looking at this and saying, "What the hell?" I get it. It's way out there, but this is the journey to transformation, the journey to enlightenment. It is not easy, but it is what you are called to be. Find the path and then be patient, be open, and be loving!

78- You Are a Snowflake

We all equally enter this life created in the image of God.

> So God created man in his own image, in the image of God He created him; Male and Female He created them.
> —Genesis 1:27

Then from the day of our birth forward, the workings of the mind and our life experiences mold us uniquely into who we perceive ourselves to be. These experiences originate from the seen and Unseen realms. The effects of the seen realm include the loving intimacy of a mother and father (hopefully), the sibling family circle, close family, our school friends, neighbors, daily work and life acquaintances, and for some, a spouse and kids of their own. The effects of the Unseen realm include our relationship with God and our Soul. All of these can impact the formation of our mind in profound and slight ways, depending on how we perceive and then integrate them into the mind.

The effects of the seen realm are relatively easy to understand compared to the infinitely complex and magical workings of the Unseen realm. The intricate web of integration of the Unseen realm into all things is gross and slight—gross in the physical realm and slight and delicate in the Unseen realm. We know we are called to journey into the Unseen realm, because when our priorities serve the material world, we experience short-term happiness followed by an empty fulfillment, and when we focus on the Unseen aspect of our life, we feel complete, whole, and purposeful. Of course, we are designed to "tune in" to the Unseen realm, but we can get disoriented if our mind is not refined enough or able to focus and concentrate. When we are not able to focus and concentrate, the noise of the seen realm will drown out our clear perception of the Unseen realm.

With time and practice we are able to "tune in" to the Unseen realm because the pathway to its realization has crystallized in our mind to show us the way whenever we choose to find God and our Soul. Even though the journey is realized, sustaining this connection is completely unique to each of us and infinitely delicate, not dissimilar to a snowflake. All snowflakes originate from a droplet of water. When the droplet freezes, it takes on a new formation. It crystallizes during descent, way above the Earth's surface, and its formation before it hits the ground is completely unique from all other snowflakes in the sky ever created.[51] This uniqueness stems from the environment that it passes through during its lifespan, and its delicate formation can be wiped away with just one touch from another object. So the next time you see a snowflake, know that your spiritual journey is similar. Your spiritual journey is crystalized deep within you, and you will have to find resilience and patience in its infinitely delicate nature, for the day that you find God's presence for even a split second is worth a lifetime of effort. Discover your crystalized pathway and find God.

79- The Horizon of the Sea

The deep blue sea is vast, mysterious, and scary, while at the same time being calm, refreshing, and peaceful. It encompasses all that the mind can see. When we stand in stillness at the edge of the ocean and peer into its infinite horizon, what we see is our home base within, our set point of the Soul. This conscious mirroring of self is essential for our spiritual growth, for it is from this self-evaluation that we realize how far off the path we have wandered.

> Because strait is the gate, and narrow is the way, which leadeth unto life, and few there be that find it. —Matthew 7:14

---

[51] National Oceanic and Atmospheric Administration, "How Do Snowflakes Form?" NOAA.gov, December 19, 2016, https://www.noaa.gov/stories/how-do-snowflakes-form-science-behind-snow

Of course, we all know that the journey takes patience and time, and if we are able to rest in this state, we will find our way, but if our immature ego mind gets too involved in what it thinks the outcome should be, we will find ourself lost. Surprisingly enough, being lost is also part of the journey, part of how God molds us into the perfect image. When we are lost, we are found, because from this vulnerable state we learn how to surrender. Our act of surrender is our gift to the world, for then we are fully participating in the Will of God. I know this seems odd to the immature ego mind, but our mature ego mind totally gets it.

80- Finding Your Joy Deep Within

When we find joy, we find contentment, and contentment helps us to rest in peace. If joy is to be found, where is it? If happiness originates in the mind, then joy originates in the heart and Soul.

> You have put more joy in my heart than they have when their grain and wine abound.
> — Psalm 4:7

Our heart and Soul are the part of us that flows into the infinite of time. The easiest way to find them within us is to quiet the mind, and the set point of our joy will be realized. When we are unable to quiet the mind, our true joy is fabricated into happiness, a temporary illusion of our joy. If you have trauma from the past, the mind might cloud your true joy with pain and suffering and cause you

148

to believe that you are unhappy, when actually, deep within, you are content and joy filled. When we are ready to flow with unfettered joy, we need to find ways to tune or refine the mind to take on the Mind of Christ. This is the journey that we were called to walk, so that we can be the example for those around us.

> "Come, follow me," Jesus said, "and I will send you out to fish for people."
> —Matthew 4:19

Yes, the journey sounds easy, but as we all know, this is a challenge in our society today. When this is the case, look for gaps in the day that you can call your own, and during this time, work to refine your mind. It starts with slowing down, being present, being still, and, from here, opening the heart to the joy within and letting it flow into every cell of your body (the Holy Spirit). Rest in the contentment of your peace within, then focus in the brain region and find Christ Consciousness or the Wisdom of God, then hold onto this state just like you loved holding onto your mother growing up! Finding this state is finding meditation or contemplation, for it is from this state that you will find your joy.

81- Blinded by the Light

What will our journey of spiritual conversion/refinement look like in our life? Will it be based on daily routine and obedience to that which we believe in, have faith in, or will we be, or maybe already have been, blinded by the light, a feeling of spiritual overwhelm? We know that St. Paul was blinded by the light for three days before he regained his sight in Damascus by Ananias.[52] Both journeys to spiritual enlightenment are perfect in the eyes of God. Whether we feel called to serve like Mother Teresa and continue to serve even when we don't feel God near,[53] or have such an overwhelming God experience that it changes the very fabric for who we think we are, like in the case of Paul, God is always right by our side, walking the journey with us, pushing us to the limit so that love is realized in this world. May love be that which we desire, and let it fill every cell of our body, for it is here that we have moved through the pain and suffering of the physical to rest in the resurrection of Christ. May this be the example for all to see where all aspects of this life can be transformed into love.

82- Where Is My AAA Route Flip Chart?

Humans have been climbing mountains for a very long time. It stems from their desire and intrigue to discover something new, something beyond their current experience. If you have ever climbed a mountain (14K'+, 6hrs+) then you know it is best to plan for the journey. You would look at the provisions needed, the best route, how technical it is, what the weather will be, and whether you are physically and mentally ready. No, you don't just start hiking blindly up the trail to the top, not prepared for what

[52] Acts 22
[53] Pascal-Emmanuel Gobry, "Mother Teresa," The Week, September 7, 2016, https://theweek.com/author/pascal-emmanuel-gobry

is just around the next turn. You determine what is needed and how you would get ready for the journey. You might find that it will take four to six months of physical training to be fully prepared, to include studying the route or alternate routes if there is a need to divert from plan A.

If you feel that you are called to walk a spiritual life, a fully awake life, then what is your plan? Have you thought about what it takes to safely navigate the road ahead? If we recognize the importance of planning for the physical/seen journey up a mountain, and we are ready to begin or are already on a spiritual journey, what are we doing to plan for this Unseen journey, a journey through the mind, a journey of refining the mind. We would need to train/practice every day and determine where we are along the journey, what the road ahead will look like, how long it will take (that's funny—we all know it will be a lifetime :-)!), and if our mind is ready for the next step or if it would be best to rest for awhile before we begin again.

If you could imagine that planning for climbing a mountain is important, navigating the refinement of the mind to realize a fully spiritual life would be like climbing ten mountains in the same day. Yes, it is a natural part of who we are and what we are called to be, and yet there is little knowledge available to show us the way to a refined mind. We have beautiful examples of the lives of Jesus, the apostles, and other spiritually minded people, and we know that there have been many examples of forty days[54] (meaning a long time) in the Bible and other references,

---

[54] "40 (number)," Wikipedia, https://en.wikipedia.org/wiki/40_(number)

so we know it will take time, but what is the exact route we will take? Where is my AAA route flip chart? We really don't have one.

The closest reference that I know of is in the Yoga Sutras,[55] four chapters each with fifty threads of thought highlighting the journey toward a refined mind. Know that the journey doesn't need to be perfect but should come with some consideration and planning. We will need to practice, learn, and then practice again. You didn't just start riding a bike; it takes time. Surrounding yourself with like-minded people is the key to a safe journey, so we don't think we are crazy half the time :-)! A fully conscious, fully refined mind is the journey toward a loving world, a joy-filled world! It starts with a daily practice and has no end! That's all it takes!

83- Bearing Your Cross

Jesus showed us that we don't need a comfortable life to live a joy-filled, loving life. A refined mind, a mature ego mind, is the first step in seeing the world through Jesus's eyes. Prior to cultivating a mature ego mind, our mind will rest in survival mode. This means it will work hard to fit into its culture at all costs. Many cultures, for many thousands of years, have outcast[56] anyone who was not normal by their standards of behavior or who didn't fit in,

---

[55] TKV Desikachar, *The Heart of Yoga: Developing a Personal Practice*, 1995

[56] "Outcast (person)," Wikipedia, https://en.wikipedia.org/wiki/Outcast_%28person%29

so this survival tactic resides deep within our DNA and is at the essence of our existence as primitive beings.

Many societies, including America, take this one step further and demand perfection—the image of perfection, the image that all is going perfect. This causes many to live a life of pretend or to work toward attaining this image of perfection. This life of pretend pushes us further from our full potential in this life and further from a resting point that is within the essence of God, Her streaming Consciousness. We are beings with limited energy, and when we place a large portion of our energy into pretending to be or trying to be something that we are not today, we will have less energy for the journey toward the Creator. Accepting who we are today is part of bearing the Cross for the day. Fully accepting every fault, blemish, and wart is our first step in putting all of our available energy into the journey that God calls us to walk. May your mind today be fully accepting and clear, lightening the load for your Journey into Consciousness.

84- Finding Your Essence

To find peace in life and peace in the moment, we will have to reduce ourselves down to our Essence (Soul). The quintessential state of all beings is when we find balance and harmony that allows the flow of Divine Energy to be free. When we find this state, we have found our foundation, and therefore anything we build on top of this foundation has the potential to be the Truth (mature ego) or illusionary (immature ego). This is why whenever we remove our illusion, we will always find clarity, euphoria, and joy. In this state we are "turned on" as instruments of God. This is our full potential in life and yet is one of our main contentions between our Soul and immature ego. This great dichotomy results in the pain and suffering that we imagine in life. Oddly enough, it is from these low places that many times we find our deepest surrender and our Essence. The greater the perceived control in life, the greater the suffering, the bigger the illusion. The larger the illusion, the greater the instability, resulting in our natural fall back into our Essence. Our nature to survive drives us to jump back on the horse to try again, resulting in our next fall. Through God's design, we have the opportunity to find our Essence around every corner, whether we fall sweetly into Her hands because of our own calculated self-surrender or tumble down from an unstable height of a castle built on illusion. Our Free Will chooses the journey. The path to God is short when we choose self-surrender. Find a meditative practice, find your Essence each day, and find your joy! It's that easy.

85- Believing in Ourself

We are intuitive beings. Our faculties to connect with God are perfectly integrated into who we are. This connection with God flows through our heart and brain so that we can feel and perceive Her in our life. When we allow God to flow through us unfettered or void of our emotions and clumsy thoughts, we are able to sense and see the beauty in Her Creation. Our training to connect begins when we are forming in our mother's womb and solidifies through the first seven years of our life. During this time we feel and see God everywhere. It is like we are completely plugged into Her Creative Flow, so that Her Divine Energy becomes a part of the fabric of who we are and what we have the potential to be later in life.

Of course, we all know what happens from seven to twenty-one years old, so let's jump ahead. Later in life we sense a calling to return home, where home is our ability to recall our first seven years of life, where our connection with God was pure, true, and complete. The reality of life is that we will be taken down many different paths from this pure connection with God. For many there will be paths where we find ourself lost in a deep, dark forest, walking aimlessly through a vast empty desert, or frightened and afraid in the abyss of the sea. This illusionary state exists because we lose the ability to BELIEVE in OURSELF. We have forgotten that within the fabric of who we are exists the key to perfect clarity. Our journey out of these places begins when we start to clean the house through picking up, putting up, and organizing our heart and mind to reduce the noise and confusion. From here it is easier to feel and see the omnipresent flow of God in every cell of our being. From here we move from being LOST to being FOUND.

> And he said to him, "Son, you are always with me, and all that is mine is yours. It was fitting to celebrate and be glad, for this your brother was dead, and is alive; he was lost, and is found."
> —Luke 15:31-32

86- More Being, Less Doing

When you feel rigid, think of all the things around you that flow. Imagine how the wind moves unseen to the eye and yet is felt on the skin, how water flows effortlessly down a creek, how a bird soars, or how a whale drifts in the water. We can learn a lot from how God's Creation naturally flows in the world.

Find a way in your day to be more present. Just "being" over "doing" is a start. We are human "beings," for goodness sake :-)! To fully surrender is to flow and to fully participate, which is completely the opposite for how our culture has molded us. How many discussions have started with, "What are you doing these days?" or, "Where do you work?" instead of, "Did you participate in God's Dance today?" Actually, maybe we should pick someone today and do exactly that :-)! Now that's some funny stuff :-)! Try it and let me know!

87- The Dance of Life

What does it mean to truly surrender? By definition, surrendering is "abandoning oneself entirely from a powerful emotion or influence." The ability to do so is at the heart of our transformation into New Life. And Jesus said to them, "You will all fall away, because it is written, 'I WILL STRIKE DOWN THE SHEPHERD, AND THE SHEEP SHALL BE SCATTERED.'"[57] To "fall away" or commit

---

[57] Mark 14:27

apostasy in Christianity is to reject Christianity when you were formerly Christian. Of course, we see this when Peter, on the night of the Last Supper, tells Jesus, "Even if all fall away, Jesus, I will not."

Yes, we all know how loyal Peter really was as he denied Jesus not once but three times in the days to come. The point here is that there is a big difference between having a desire to surrender and actually surrendering. If Peter had truly surrendered, he would have confirmed when asked that indeed he was with Jesus and then probably would have been on the Cross with him, but he was not ready for that level of surrender. Peter began his journey of transformation in the years to come and did die for Jesus in the long run.

When our mind takes on Christ Consciousness and our heart is open to the Holy Spirit, our journey of surrender will begin. Slow and steady is our path to transformation. Don't make it a race like our culture loves to turn everything into. It starts with your next breath and the realization that your life is a gift and then stopping to listen to the whisper deep within to see how your actions today are to align with the Dance of Life!

88- New Humans from a New Earth

When you look at planet Earth, do you see an object or a living organism? Is the Earth alive, or is it just a big round marble hurtling through space? I'm sure if you are reading this, then you see an alive Earth, Mother Earth, which has been hosting human life for over two hundred thousand years.

Science has been measuring the frequencies of objects for a long time, to include the frequency of the Earth. This frequency is called the Schumann Resonance and is equivalent to the heartbeat for Mother Earth. The Earth's Heartbeat has been steady at 7.83Hz ever since 2014 when it began to accelerate to somewhere in the 15 to 25 Hz range, and on January 31, 2016, it reached frequencies of 36+ for the first time in recorded history.[58] This change is incredible, a phenomenon, not dissimilar to the 2012 phenomenon highlighting the end of the Mayan calendar and the beginning of transformative events on earth.[59]

Do these changes impact us? They sure do. When we are being formed in our mother's womb, the frequencies around us impact our biochemistry to include our brain and ultimately our DNA. The newness of Mother Earth's frequency is creating the new humans of our day. This higher frequency gives rise to higher states of Consciousness for all living things and has a profound impact on things and people that are born into it. How do we prepare the way for the new human? For those that are already conscious and are working to find stillness every day and in this stillness a Union with God, you are

[58] Carol Mann, "COSMIC CAFE: Earth's Accelerating Vibration," Buckrail, February 15, 2017,
https://buckrail.com/cosmic-cafe-earths-accelerating-vibration/
[59] "2012 phenomenon" Wikipedia,
https://en.wikipedia.org/wiki/2012_phenomenon

already doing your part. We are called to be loving examples for others, so that from our example more can see the path to love.

89- The End of Monday Night Football

There are 228,450 known species in the ocean and as many as 2 million more that remain a total mystery. The number of species alive on Earth is 8.7 million eukaryotic species (cell-based organisms) give or take 1.3 million, with 80 percent believed to still be undiscovered.[60] Yes, stop wondering what an alien from another world would look like—they would probably look like a version of what we already have here on Earth :-)!

When we look at the animal kingdom through our mind's eye, we see birds that make us feel light, open, and expansive; dolphins that make us feel happy, flowing, and free; and snakes that make us want to get up and run. Why do we have such a vast range of feelings for different species? Are these feelings embedded in our DNA for survival purposes, do we have a past experience, or does our mind create scenarios that cause the feelings? I can only imagine that it is very complex, maybe some, all, or more than we can imagine. I get it—we are emotional beings. By God's design our emotions have been stirring up our actions way before we were conscious (Adam & Eve) for survival purposes, and this was a "good thing."

---

[60] Lee Sweetlove, "Number of Species on Earth Tagged at 8.7 Million," Nature.com, August 23, 2011, https://www.nature.com/articles/news.2011.498

For sure, we are all called to have higher conscious actions, loving actions, and less emotional actions, reactive actions. I'm grateful that by the Grace of God we are all being led down a path of Consciousness, but if we were to gauge where we are on this path of conversion as a society, I would have to say that it is going to be a long road. In the meantime, we will need to find endless patience, forgiveness, humility, compassion, and love for ourself and others. Let us deep dive into where we are in this transformation as human beings. Survival is all about winning and losing. If a tiger enters the room, your instinct is to survive, no question about it. We are geared to our core for winning and losing, and no one knows this better than men. They have been fighting battles for the last two hundred thousand plus years and maybe even got good at it. Now in the last two thousand years we have been called to take off the battle gear and believe that there is nothing to fear and that it is time to surrender. Yeah right?!

As we see in society today there are many emotions for one another. These emotions again are very complex just like our animal example, but even more so because of our competitive nature. Here begins our challenge, "You must die to self to find yourself."[61] It will take time, but we will be moving in the right direction when more people are excited to be gathering for spiritually conscious reasons over competitive ones. Yes, when there is no longer Monday Night Football :-), we will be getting closer. In the meantime, the job for the rest of us is about being patient

---

[61] John 3:30

160

and an example for what it means to be consciously loving. Share your love for another today and watch the ripple of your love flow beautifully into the world.

90- Haiti's Earthquake

Jesus's journey of forty days and forty nights shows us that to live fully awake as an instrument of God, a major transformation will take place over time. This transformation is all about learning how to fully participate in the Dynamic Flow of Divinity. The journey will take us out of the bondage of our nature (satan) and into a new life that is one with the Creator. This lowercase use of *satan* represents our own inner struggle for how an immature ego will set up roadblocks, create distracting desires, or cause us to think that being busy means we have purpose, and therefore holding us back from walking a path of transformation. When we are ready to begin this journey, we need to cultivate clarity in the mind. This clarity is like seeing life through a new lens that helps us to see the true workings of God.

As an example, our nature sees the earthquake in Haiti as a terrible thing for the people of Haiti. This force of nature destroyed the city of Port-au-Prince, affecting 3 million people and killing 230,000. Through another lens, maybe each of those Haitian Souls affected signed up to be a part of this event because the outcome would result in something bigger. Their Souls fully surrendered and had Faith in God. The result was World Compassion, and the experience for many was of love for someone they didn't even know physically through an experience of true communion with another.

Our journey of transformation is complicated, and not really what we think it is. If we were to look at our spiritual transformation visually in a chart, using the y-axis as a measure of our desire to grow spiritually and the x-axis as our actual spiritual growth, then over time this chart would turn into an asymptote graph that grows exponentially with time based on our mental desire to grow spiritually, meaning that our journey would take an infinite amount of mental desire to get to our endpoint. On the other hand if we are able to surrender into God's transformation for us like the Souls in Haiti, it is effortless.

What does this even mean? It means that the only thing holding us back from being beautifully loving beings, Christ-Like, is that we haven't learned how to tame our nature, release our control, and refine the perceived pain and suffering of our immature ego mind, so that what remains is the unfettered streaming flow of Divinity within a highly stable human instrument. Our journey of transformation begins in the mind, the Breathe Pillar, and is directly impacted by how we Eat, Move, and Sleep.

91- Taking on the Pain of Another

A spiritually minded world (Christ Consciousness) will be realized when the human race learns to have compassion and love for one another. To begin the journey, a person will need to develop the faculty of connecting with another. It starts with connecting physically and being present with another regardless of anything that drives you crazy about them :-), yes, to truly and fully accept the other with all of their baggage, faults, warts, and wounds. This is just the start. The next step is the beginning of new faculties for many, which is the ability to connect with another spiritually, or to be in communion with another. This is a natural part of who we are as God's Instruments, but being conscious of it is where we are called to go.

Being conscious of this will take time. The journey is accelerated through a practice of stillness, concentration, and ultimately meditation. For it is through meditation that we begin to experience the union of all, a non-dual Universe where all is one. Meditation teaches us how to find the whisper of God within, the streaming Consciousness of all that is seen (4 percent) and Unseen (96 percent) in the Universe. Over time we will be able to stay connected with the whisper even during days when the mental stimulation of our senses begins to drown out the whisper, because we have mastered concentration. Now we are moving in the right direction to be spiritually connected with another.

When we are in communion with another and recognize their physical, mental, and spiritual limitations, this is true compassion. The feeling of compassion comes from their heart center to ours, allowing the person or groups of people to release some of their suffering and limitations through the one that has opened their heart for them. It is through the work of God that the suffering of one can be released through another. Take Jesus, for example. His compassion and love for us relieved us of our sufferings and is still at work today! Find time to be still every day, so that the mind can slow down and you can begin to see the workings of God around you. Develop a mind that is able to concentrate and have love for God. Once you are able to do these two things and have a daily meditation practice, you will be stepping closer to your full potential as an instrument of God's making. Be still, Be Focused, and See God!

92- Relationships 101

God's Creation is all about bringing things together. Let's start small. When you place two hydrogen molecules and one oxygen molecule near each other at the right temperature and pressure, they will want to form a relationship, a bond, and this relationship gives us life, water. The expansion of God's Creation is about bringing things together to make 1 + 1 equal 4 or 6. It's not a linear expansion, it's a rapid one.

Let's just say for the fun of it that atoms have Consciousness and even a personality, what would they be saying? Are they excited to find the other element in space and time and eager to bond, but after a period of time they get tired of the other :-)? You probably see where I'm going with this. Yes, all things are called to find relationships in the Universe. From the smallest of small things to the Earth and the Moon and as humans, we all have relationships with one another. If at the Unseen level we are all super connected, why do we need physical relationships to facilitate the production of a better version of ourself? Maybe because we are not at an endpoint, not stable, not fully ready to transform the flow of Divine Energy within ourselves, but together able to find the best next step in time for manifesting God's Creation.

Where are these communal relationships? They start with the Family 101 class and our parents, the function of dysfunction, the molding of our version 1.0. Here we learn to be loved and to love. We realize that we can depend on another to give us what we need and not always what we want. These bonds drive us crazy :-) and we learn the need for independence and the difficulties in breaking or finding distance in our relationships. Somewhere in there we take the class Friends 101. We experience the fun of being with others who are not trying to mold us and accept us for who we are. We find that they are great sounding boards as we work to find ourself. We learn to forgive and to accept another for who they are. We recognize that no one is perfect and that we all have limitations and faults.

Then there is First Love 101. Your heart center gets turned on and you experience your second deep intimate connection with another after your mother. This new super-high-frequency bond is something you have never experienced before. This experience lasts for a while and then dulls down to a level that the body is able to maintain over time, and we learn what it means to be in communion with another.

We cycle back through all of these a few times and hopefully at some point find ourselves taking 400 level classes and knowing that we will be in school our whole life :-). At the 400 level classes we see how intricate relationships are, because the human instrument is intricate, and if we want to remain in communion with others, which is what God calls us to do, we will have to work at it. Our ultimate potential is when we master patience, compassion, humility, and intimacy to realize the highest state of love for another, Agape! This is the highest and purest form of love for another, where 1 + 1 always equals a very large number.

93- Seeing with New Eyes

Our world is not what we perceive it to be. It is much more. Yes, we have these wonderful eyes that allow us to see the world around us, and yet with them we only see vibrations from 380 to 700 nanometers[62], while the vibrations in the Universe range from 1 hertz to 10^{25} hertz[63]. Yes, that means that there are some wavelengths the size of atoms. Therefore, we are only able to perceive 3.2×10^{-12} percent or 0.0000000000032 percent of the Universe with our eyes. The rest is perceived with some

---

[62] Source: https://science.nasa.gov, Visible Light, Science Mission Directorate
[63] Source: https://en.wikipedia.org, Electromagnetic Spectrum

other faculty outside of our senses. At a very high level we call this faculty our *consciousness*.

For many years, Humans have been working to refine their understanding of their Consciousness into Higher Consciousness, God Consciousness, Yahweh, The Holy Spirit, Christ Consciousness, Mother Mary, Prana, The Buddha, Brahma, Vishnu, Shiva, Allah, The Great Spirit, etc. We naturally have a desire to share this profound new Knowing of refined Consciousness with others. This is a beautiful thing, but when a person is still in their survival gear or predominately remains in an immature ego state, their sharing of this Knowing can be clumsy, not understood by others, or downright nonproductive. Of course, Jesus shared this with many people, "Go and tell no one."[64] Therefore our relationship with the Father should, for the most part, remain in Secret until the day that we Awaken into Full Consciousness through experiencing a personal Presence with God.

94- Keeping an Eye on Your Speed

Of course when we talk about stillness, we generally think about stilling the mind and from this stillness finding the inner voice of God, but have you ever thought about how fast you are moving when you are sitting still? Let's have some fun with this one :-)! Let's start with our daily motion. The Earth rotates on its axis every twenty-four hours, so a point near the equator must move close to 1,000 miles per hour to complete its rotation in a day. As

---

[64] Matthew 8:4

you move north or south from the Equator, the speed slows, which is why we have wind and currents in the world. On a yearly basis the Earth revolves around the Sun every 365 days at a distance of about 93 million miles. The path of the Earth's orbit is close to 600 million miles long, so we have to travel about 43,000 miles per hour to complete our journey in a year.

Now comes the tricky part, measuring the Sun's motion. It is tricky because there is no reference point. Every star in the Universe has its own motion. They are either expanding from one another or rotating around the other, not to mention that quantum physics has now proven that space is also expanding—weird, right? Think of it this way: a square inch a second ago is now two square inches :-). Don't think too long about this topic unless you are ready for your head to spin! Back to our linear world. Let's look at how fast we are moving within the Milky Way. It takes the Sun about 225 million years to complete one rotation around our galaxy. That's about twenty galactic years since the Earth and Sun have formed. To complete this rotation in one galactic year, we are traveling about 483,000 miles per hour. This is a super-fast speed. The speed of light travels at an incomprehensible speed of 670 million miles per hour.

Now comes the super-weird stuff. From the Big Bang, we have physical things moving outward and also space expanding, which has the Milky Way Galaxy moving at an astounding 1.3 million miles per hour. So just when you thought you haven't done much today, know that you are moving in all kinds of directions[65].

95- Molding the Mind to See Consciousness

When we become conscious of God, there is a Knowing in the mind and a Knowing in the heart, and the latter is part of our instinct and an easier path if our mind is not ready. The mind is not ready when the senses, concentration, or meditation have not been mastered. For many this is a lifelong journey of practice with an occasional experience with the "Big Guy" :-)! When the Knowing is from the heart, we feel the presence of God through our body. This type of Knowing is void from the noise of the mind, so we are able to have a purely unfettered experience of the flow of Consciousness. This is probably how much of the animal kingdom experiences God. Mankind evolved beyond this with Adam and Eve or our mental Consciousness of God. As we start to mold this Consciousness within the ego, there are two ways to go: the development of a mature ego or an immature ego. The mature ego mind sees a non-dual existence of all, meaning that God is all—everything—and an immature ego mind will perceive a dualistic world where God is over there and we are over here. For me, I bounce around between a mature and immature ego, but consciously work to realize a non-dual world where the presence and love of God is everywhere.

---

[65] www.nightsky.jpl.nasa.gov, The Universe in the Classroom, No. 71 Spring 2007, by Andrew Franknoi

96- Ask a Tree

Imagine an infinite sea of God Consciousness in our Universe, of which 96 percent is Unseen and unmeasurable, called the spiritual realm, and the other 4 percent is the physical realm. Within this physical realm we appear unique and individual and yet are completely integrated at the spiritual realm or into the sea of God Consciousness. Do you need a brain to have God Consciousness? Ask a tree! I hate to say it, but there might be some trees that have a higher Consciousness than some people on this earth. And again it looks like we are all physically separate, the trees and the people, and yet we are more connected than we realize.

97- Directing the Mind

Yoga helps us along this journey of forming the mind, so that God can flow easily through the body. At a basic level, it helps us remove soreness and dis-ease from the body and strengthen the muscles to properly support our skeletal system, but ultimately it is designed to help us refine the mind so it can accept the powerful flow of God and remain stable. Yes, Consciousness is growing and expanding whether we like it or not, which is probably why we see so many people with behavioral health conditions today. As God evolves Her Creation and turns up Consciousness and our minds are not ready for it, mental instability will continue to grow.

So how does yoga help this? First and foremost the mind must know how to concentrate. "Yoga is the ability to direct the mind exclusively toward an object and sustain that direction without any distractions" (Yoga Sutra 1.2). Of course, all of us today would read that sentence and think, "Yeah right? Good luck with that :-)." Yes, we have way too many distractions and too much business today, not to mention that many haven't found their purpose and believe that being busy is the solution. Start with a daily practice and begin to walk a path of loving Consciousness, the path that Jesus called us to walk.

98- Dancing with the Creator

Is it more important for your mind to know your purpose in life or to be present with the flow of the Creator as life unfolds? Both, we must search for our purpose each day and then flow day-to-day with the infinitely dynamic Creation of God.

"Be Still And Know That I Am God", is a powerful way to begin the journey of flowing with God's infinitely dynamic Creation. This stillness will lead us into consciousness when the mind is healthy. There are many factors that affect the health of our mind to include what we eat, our environment, past experiences, our genetics, and so forth, and it is our responsibility to assess the hygiene of our mind and find ways to maintain its health, so that our Dance with the Creator aligns step-by-step.

99- Just a Little Bit of Good

A daily practice of yoga, or knowing the importance of the body, mind, and Soul connection and maintaining the human instrument in harmony, is the first step in building the stability needed to grow spiritually. Yes, a daily practice is just a minimum, because there is much work to be done. We are in the middle of God's Creation, not at the endpoint. As an example, consider how much the human race today is more Christlike. Are there still more ways for people to be more patient, forgiving, compassionate, and loving? Just looking at myself, I practice yoga every day and realize that it will take all the days of my life just to appear as the shadow of Christ. So many may ask, "Then why even try?" The answer is that through communion, when one learns, all learn. Yes, we are all super connected in the Unseen realm. There is no individual. Every little bit of good that you do in this physical world, even unknown to other physical people, is integrated fully into the collective Consciousness of God's Creation. So go out and do some good today and believe that it will be known by all!

100- A Practice Opens the Lotus Flower

A long-term practice of meditation steers the practitioner toward a life of contemplation, a life that is integrated at some level into the Unseen realm. This life is revealed because during the initial stages of meditation, the mind slowly refines so that it can begin to perceive the Unseen world that it is immersed in. Cultivating these new

172

faculties is like learning to hear someone whisper at a rock concert. You would probably have to learn to read lips and possibly refine how your mind processes the vibrations you hear so you could focus only on the vibrations coming from the person doing the whispering. If this sounds complex or probably impossible, then I have provided a good example :-), because to attune to the Unseen realm is very complex and yet a part of our design.

We are designed to tune into the Unseen realm because we are designed to tune into the Creator. Make no mistake about it, the process of refining the mind will, many times, leave one confused, afraid, alone, and in a state of disbelief. That is why this journey is definitely easier if traveled with someone who has a meditation practice or is on a contemplative journey themselves. Just know that the longer you stay on the path, the more peace, joy, and love you will realize. This is the beginning of the opening up of the lotus flower, of birth, and of awakening. Your life is now "A New Life" and one to explore for the rest of your physical days.

101- Be a Rubber Band

A conscious life is a dynamic dance. An organic flow of stillness and movement that form us into who we are today and who we will be in the future. If we stay in the flow life will appear simple, effortless, and joy filled, but if we believe that we have personal control over this dynamic dance then life will appear difficult, challenging, and/or tense. This dichotomy is part of our total life experience. It is when we realize that it is not personal that we begin to again flow with the dance. A rubber band probably has a better chance of accepting its resting and tension states than many people do in accepting these states in their lives, but as we mature the ego and begin to soften the edges of our perceived control it will help us to integrate naturally into God's beautiful dynamic dance.

102- Live Life Fully Awake

Don't avoid your fears, embrace them. They are woven deep into the fabric of our existence, so to deny them would be to deny who you are. When we run from the sheer nakedness of who we really are, we begin an illusion of pretending. American culture and many others have capitalized off of the desires of many on the Earth to live a life of pretend. This desire is quenched in the TV programs, news, and movies we watch, the material items we buy, and the false power we feel from a work title we might have. An immature ego loves to participate in this pretend world, a world that ultimately deepens the illusion, deceit, pain, and suffering that we feel.

If unconscious of the path we are on, we can spiral into a dark abyss, or for many today, behavioral health issues. To embrace your fear means to be humble, forgiving, and loving. This path shows us how to transform our fears, not transmit them. Through this we begin a journey of molding our ego into a mature state that helps us walk a spiritual life, a real life, a conscious life. We are already just a super-tiny fraction of God's existence. There is no need to make ourselves bigger than God expects. Finding our tiny self, including our fears in this big world and infinitely large universe, might take a lifetime, but in the end will afford us more peace, joy, and love than our hearts and minds can imagine. Find a mature ego, remove your illusion, and live life fully awake!

103- God Is in the Gap

For many, it is known that God has called us to serve through our actions. This participation is the accumulation of all of our conscious moments in time, which add up to our purpose. This is our ultimate calling in the universe, and God rewards us through a Knowing in our heart and mind every time we align just a little bit with God's Will. If we want to deepen our purpose, we will have to find the gaps in time.

In 1915 Albert Einstein determined in his theory of general relativity that time was not what we imagine it to be. He found that depending on the relative speed of one object to another, the duration of time changed. The faster you physically move, the slower time becomes relative to another object moving at a slower speed. Now this is just an example of one object to another, so you could imagine how complicated calculating time would be if there were billions of objects all moving at various speeds all across the universe. Just to confuse the matter even more, Hubble and the age of quantum physics are now showing that galaxies are moving away from each other faster than the speed of light — that the physical objects aren't the only thing expanding from one another, that space itself is also expanding.[66]

Now, I don't know if everyone needs to understand this to see my next point, which is that being conscious means finding liminal space, the time between moments in time, the moment when time almost stops relative to everyone else in the world. I can imagine that it happens to us unconsciously all the time, or consciously during our meditation or contemplation practices. The point is that to begin to understand the working of God and how we can fully participate in the Will of God, we have to move beyond the physical, because God has placed the Knowing between every moment of our physical life. Finding God means being still relative to everything else and then seeing the space between time, the gap, the liminal space. So take time today to find your gap, and in it total Consciousness.

104- Finding Our New Form

How interesting that to truly find yourself, you have to be really good at losing yourself.

> Whoever finds their life will lose it, and whoever loses their life for my sake will find it.
> —Matthew 10:39

---

[66] Fraser Cain, "How Can Galaxies Recede Faster Than the Speed of Light?" Universe Today, 2015, https://www.universetoday.com/13808/how-can-galaxies-recede-faster-than-the-speed-of-light/

Therefore, if anyone is in Christ, the new creation has come: The old has gone, the new is here.
—II Corinthians 5:17

Let's just start with something very apparent. Our brain and hence our mind are not capable of clearly seeing all of God's Creation. We are just a sliver of the Creation with limited to no control over the Will of God, nor Her natural outpouring. At best we have the opportunity to participate in Creation, if and when we are able to tune into how our actions can best align. For many it is done unconsciously, and for a few it is conscious, because they have found their purpose in this life, how their puzzle piece fits perfectly into the complexities of the workings of our Creator. How do we find our purpose, allowing us to be in harmony with God's Will? This sounds easy, but until we mature our ego, this journey will seem like nothing but a struggle, a burden, and an inconvenience. How do we begin this journey? It takes practice, a practice that helps us to find the union, clarity, and love of our Creator, and from this connection a personal will to lose ourself, to find the gift that God has so perfectly placed in our lap.

If we could all flow like water in this life, our lives would be effortless, simple, and joy filled. A water molecule doesn't really know where it is going nor even care. It is happy to be in communion with other water molecules, so that it can flow so beautifully. It was created as an instrument of God to fulfill Her plan. It does not ask God, "Why did we turn this way in the stream, or why do you tear me apart at high temperatures?" No, it just fully participates in the plan without question, because it accepts the plan that God has Created.

> This is the day the LORD has made. We will rejoice and be glad in it.
> —Psalm 118:24

In an ideal upbringing an individual is surrounded with faith, hope, and love. This helps one to walk a life of compassion, forgiveness, joy, and love. You could imagine in this state that our mind would be molded into a mature state that integrates one into a state of communion with all beings, allowing them to easily remain in this beautiful state of higher Consciousness—a state where the natural instincts of our primitive self, our primitive existence are able to remain quiet and still. In the absence of this unrealistic perfect upbringing :-), one realizes this mature state when they are able to see who they are in the world. This realization is called the ego, or the point in time at which Adam and Eve realized their existence, their Consciousness, and their nakedness. Since it was important for God to design us to first survive, so that we could see a day of Consciousness, we will have to work to form and mold the mind into this state of maturity. It is easy to know how mature your ego is by how many times it takes offense in a day. When we are not offended by the actions of others, then our ego is mature, but if we take offense or get upset by the actions of others, then there is an opportunity to improve. If we are being honest, we will all work at this our whole life. We will drift in and out of this conscious journey, but just know that every little bit of work moves us closer to the Will of God.

105- Get on, It's a Free Ride

All beings with a Consciousness have the ability to perceive and integrate into the workings of Creation. Our existence spans between the Unseen and seen realms, where the Unseen realm makes up most of our existence. Quantum physics has already proven that 96 percent of the energy in the universe is Unseen and unmeasurable, leaving 4 percent of our energy to reside in the physical world. For many human beings, their mind sees the seen realm as 100 percent of their existence, and yet in reality it is just a tiny part. Since the Creator is around us and in us always, we are afforded the opportunity to see clearly the workings of the Creator, if we choose. This happens when our mind is calm, steady, and accepting and we fall into a deep state of surrender.

If we are able to maintain this state for a period of time, the illusion of the seen realm is lifted and we begin to realize that there is something more, something beautiful. This Knowing intrigues us to continue the journey, which turns into our spiritual growth. If we remain on this path, our spirituality matures, and the clarity of the unknown is enhanced, allowing our actions to align with the natural outpouring of the Creator. Since the Creator has placed us in communion with one another in the Unseen state, what one Soul learns, the others can access, so know that as you work toward maturing spiritually, your work is helping all of Creation. We do not walk this journey alone. It is one journey for all of Creation. Find ways to mature spiritually every day. If you are reading this, then you know the journey takes a lifetime, but time to the Creator is not what we think it is, so just sit back and enjoy the FREE ride while it is here with the ticket of Grace that the Creator has so lovingly provided.

106- We are the Lightbulb

The Force of Electricity when applied to a lightbulb creates the action of light, so too does the Force of The Holy Spirit (Prakriti) when applied to the Soul (Atman) of a surrendered or liberated human mind create loving actions on this Earth. Yes a surrendered mind is a pure mind and the actions of a pure mind will always align with the Will of God (Brahman). To achieve this state we will first have to find and hold a mature ego mind, because from this perspective it is easier to see the Glory of the God.

107- Yoga Accelerates God's Vision

In the future an individual's True Wealth will not be measured by how much money they have, but by the number of good deeds they complete in their life. The Soul is constantly working to move the physical instrument into this perfect form, but is dampened by the nature of the body's quest to survive amidst a perfectly safe environment. The techniques of yoga have the ability to accelerate the Souls pursuit of molding the physical form, so that the Will of God may be realized.

108- Participating in Consciousness

Start with an endless space filled with your most beautifully conceived white light vibrating with pure love super connected with itself. Call that which fills this space Higher Consciousness (God). This Consciousness is expanding and growing at all times per its own Will in multiple dimensions. It takes all that is known and experienced in this moment to design a path that fulfills Its Will in the next moment in time.

Where is the human experience in this model? Imagine within this Higher Consciousness space a temporary shell that is formed around a tiny piece of Higher Consciousness. The shell represents our human experience and the tiny piece of Higher Consciousness, within the shell, our Soul. The formation of the shell by the Higher Consciousness is the formation of a new dimension that we call the Universe or more specifically the human experience. All that is perceived and learned within this human experience is shared instantly with the Higher Consciousness and all other humans.

When this individual human experience is created, the thickness of the shell (ego) is very thin so all experiences outside the shell can continue to easily flow to the Consciousness within. With time, the ego is formed, for survival purposes, and the thickness of the shell grows, creating an illusion of space between us and God Consciousness. For some, the shell's thickness naturally recedes over time to a thin state again. The rate of this thinning is proportional to the human's willingness to focus all of their desires toward reconnecting with God. In the end the shell is once again reduced to nothingness, so that all that was learned/experienced remains infinitely within Higher Consciousness.

Could our Earthly Experiences be used to facilitate other formations of human experiences on the other side of the universe? You already know the answer :-).

Appendix

2 to 1 Breathing Exercise

Sit down with your spine upright or lying, close your eyes and focus on the breath in and out through the nose. Use Ujjayi Breathing to steady and slow the breath if you choose. Create a slow smooth rhythm for a few breaths, then begin to lengthen the exhale while maintaining the length of the inhale. You can use counting to assist you. Work up to an inhale for 4 seconds and an exhale for 8 seconds. Practice this for at least 3 minutes each day or as needed to calm the mind and body.

This breathing exercise tips the nervous system from the sympathetic (fight, flight, freeze) mode to the parasympathetic (calm, digestive, healing) mode of the body and can be used to help you fall asleep or relax if you feel anxious.

Ujjayi Breathing Exercise

Sit down with your spine upright or lying, close your eyes and focus on the breath in and out through the nose. Begin to make an "Ocean Sound" with your breath through constricting the vocal cords to narrow the gap that the breath can move through. Allow the mind to focus on the gentle sound and vibration that you created for at least 3 minutes.

This breathing exercise activates concentration to help bring the mind into the moment and the Vagus Nerve, the main nerves of the parasympathetic nervous system that control digestion, heart rate, and the immune system.

Four Pillars of Optimal Health

The Four Pillars of Optimal Health was developed by Dr. Amy to help her patients progress toward their highest level of optimal living. Because patient compliance with lifestyle change can be challenging, she knew that the Pillars needed to be Reliable, Available, and Doable (RAD) leading her to develop the following stages toward optimal living.

Note: If you have pre-existing conditions, consult your provider before changing your existing care plan.

❖ Phase I, Learning the Basics
  ➢ Breathe- 2 minutes of stillness per day
  ➢ Eat- Eliminate added sugars/sweeteners, eliminate processed foods, add more plant rich foods
  ➢ Move- 14 minutes of movement per day
  ➢ Sleep- At least 7 hrs per night

❖ Phase II, Integrating the Basics
  ➢ Breathe- Learn the Body, Mind, and Soul Connection, 10 minutes of meditation per day
  ➢ Eat- In addition to Phase 1, optimize macronutrients, micronutrients, fiber, and fluids by including 5-7 fruits & vegetables per day, optimal fats, optimal protein, and water with each meal.
  ➢ Move- 14 minutes of target heart rate per day
  ➢ Sleep- 7-8 hrs per night

❖ Phase III, Optimizing Life

- ➤ Breathe- 20 minutes of moving meditation and 20 minutes of still meditation per day
- ➤ Eat- In addition to Phase 2, include 7+ vegetables per day, 2-3 fruits per day, "Test Don't Guess"- perform nutrient analysis, food sensitivity and gut testing to optimize your personal nutrition plan
- ➤ Move- 20 minutes of target heart rate, 10 minutes of strengthening, and 10 minutes of stretching per day
- ➤ Sleep- 7-9 hrs per night of restful sleep

If you are ready to begin or rekindle your path into optimal living and would like a virtual guide to help you graduate Phase I of Dr. Amy's Four Pillars of Optimal Health, please goto www.opt2livcourses.com and choose our OPT2CHANGE 21 Day Wellness Program.

Four Pillars Worksheet

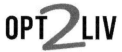

Journal

Day 1 2 3 4 5 6 7

Weekly Focus
Eat Colors of Rainbow

Participant Name _____ *Date* _____

Eat Times	Food & Drink Intake (include type, amount, brand)	Macronutrients & Micronutrients
Waking		Servings P ___ Servings F ___ Servings C ___ # Different Colors of Rainbow _____
Breakfast		Servings P ___ Servings F ___ Servings C ___ # Different Colors of Rainbow _____
Mid-AM Snack		Servings P ___ Servings F ___ Servings C ___ # Different Colors of Rainbow _____
Lunch		Servings P ___ Servings F ___ Servings C ___ # Different Colors of Rainbow _____
Mid-PM Snack		Servings P ___ Servings F ___ Servings C ___ # Different Colors of Rainbow _____
Dinner		Servings P ___ Servings F ___ Servings C ___ # Different Colors of Rainbow _____
PM Snack		Servings P ___ Servings F ___ Servings C ___ # Different Colors of Rainbow _____

P-Protein, F-Fat, C-Carbohydrate

Breathe	Move	Sleep	Social
Stress reduction practices:	Type, Time, Intensity Aerobic: Strength: Flexibility:	Hours: In Bed __ hrs, Asleep __ hrs Quality: ___ Poor ___Fair ___Good Rested after Sleep? Y or N	Supporting: Non-Supporting:
Stressors:			

Personal Meditation Practice

My morning meditation practice began when I was 10 years old and has evolved into the following practice. It consists of 20 minutes of a moving meditation followed by 20 minutes of still meditation, and serves as a means to prepare my body and mind to flow with the Spirit and God's Infinite Grace:

- ❖ Contemplation/Meditation Preparation
    - ➤ Start the meditation app Insight Timer
    - ➤ Place meditation blanket
    - ➤ Light a candle
    - ➤ Place a Crucifix at the top of the blanket, obviously optional :-)
- ❖ Centering
    - ➤ Sit in a Hero (Virasana) position
    - ➤ Repeatedly exhale through the mouth to soften the emotional body
    - ➤ Find your base bandhas to begin Prana Vayu movement upward into the brain region
    - ➤ Use ujjayi breathing to inhale energy up from the base of the spine to the heart and exhale from the heart out the crown of the head to the heavens, until the flow of Prana/divine energy is realized, then make the sign of the cross
    - ➤ Pray the Nicene Creed, Our Father, Hail Mary, and Glory Be
    - ➤ Bow (Child Pose, Balasana) with the intention of surrendering the physical to the Soul
    - ➤ Pray Come Holy Spirit

- Inhale up through the nose, lifting the arms, palms, and chin to the heavens, exhale through the mouth while lowering the arms and chin
- Be still
- Moving meditation to deepen my understanding of how the mind can surrender to the body. Each pose is held for 30 seconds, 5 breaths, or a Come Holy Spirit prayer
  - Forward fold (Paschimottanasana)
  - Seated angle (Upavistha Konasana)
  - Double pigeon (Agnistambhasana)
  - Half lotus head to knee
  - Seated twist (Sage Bharadvaj, Bharadvajasana)
  - Hidden lotus, hands on crucifix
  - Sphinx hidden lotus
  - Pull knees in, kiss feet of Jesus
  - Press back into lotus forward fold
  - Change lotus position of legs
- Reiki
  - Use Palm Chakras to remove congestion from chakras. With palms facing down, begin with one hand in front of the face, moving downward. When at bottom, place the other hand in front of the face, moving downward. Begin a circular movement with the hands, inhaling for four quick breaths, then exhaling for four quick breaths. Repeat.
- Kriya
  - Kapalbhati, 108 rounds
  - Agnisar Kriya, 54 rounds, leaning forward

- ➤ Lift up into Rising Lotus and say Come Holy Spirit (I generally get a massive amount of energy flowing up from this process.)
- ❖ Pranayama
  - ➤ Alternate nostril breathing (Anuloma Viloma),
    - ■ 3 Rounds
      - • Inhale left side, pray Come Holy Spirit, first round said once, second round said twice and so on
      - • Inhale right side, chant Om Namo Bhagavate Vasudevaya, first round said three times, second round said six times and so on
- ❖ Still Meditation/Contemplation
  - ➤ Centering
    - ■ Light incense, blow out, and then write in the air one Om and three crosses
    - ■ Get into lotus position
    - ■ Engage lower bandhas, and tune into the movement of divine energy within (Prana, Holy Spirit, Chi, etc.) and direct it upward into the brain region (Ajna or Sahasrara Chakra)
    - ■ Surrender the physical to the Soul and divine energy
    - ■ Visualize a glow from the inside out, allowing all cells to witness the vibration of Love
    - ■ Visualize all family members in a circle, also realizing the flow of divine energy from the core of their being out in all directions
    - ■ Placing all of us in the beautiful glow of divine love, wait for the Holy Spirit or the Grace of

God to touch this intention. When this happens, allow this divine glow to extend all the way out to the edge of the universe, pushing out any vibration that isn't needed, and as this sphere of divine love begins to contract, imagine that it makes a copy of all that is good in the universe all the way back to this beautiful glowing sphere surrounding the family and me.
- Visualize a mirror image of each child, one facing toward the center of the circle and the other facing outward toward their significant other to form their own circle of light.
- Release this intention to the universe
➢ Still meditation
- Focus up into the brain region
- Look in the direction of God to allow divine energy to paint images of higher Consciousness

Prayer/Mantra Reference

❖ Nicene Creed
  ➢ We believe in one God, the Father, the Almighty, Maker of Heaven and Earth, of all things visible and invisible. We believe in Jesus Christ, His only Son, our Lord, who was born of the Virgin Mary, suffered under Pontius Pilot, crucified, died, and was buried. On the third day, He rose again in fulfillment of the scriptures. He ascended into heaven and is seated at the right hand of the Father, and his Kingdom will have no end. We believe in the Holy

Spirit, the holy Catholic Church, the communion of Saints, the forgiveness of sins, the resurrection of the body, and life everlasting. Amen.

- ❖ Our Father
  - ➢ Our Father, Who art in heaven, hallowed be Thy name; Thy kingdom come; Thy will be done on earth as it is in heaven. Give us this day our daily bread; and forgive us our trespasses as we forgive those who trespass against us; and lead us not into temptation, but deliver us from evil. Amen.
- ❖ Hail Mary
  - ➢ Hail Mary, full of grace. The Lord is with thee. Blessed art thou amongst women, and blessed is the fruit of thy womb, Jesus. Holy Mary, Mother of God, pray for us sinners, now and at the hour of our death. Amen.
- ❖ Glory Be
  - ➢ Glory be to the Father, and to the Son, and to the Holy Spirit, as it was in the beginning, is now, and ever shall be, world without end. Amen.
- ❖ Come Holy Spirit
  - ➢ Come, Holy Spirit, fill the hearts of us your faithful and kindle in us the fire of your love. Send forth your Spirit, and we shall be created, and You shall renew the face of the earth. O, God, who by the light of the Holy Spirit, instructs the hearts of the faithful, grants that by the same Holy Spirit we may

be truly wise and ever rejoice in His consolations. Through Christ Our Lord. Amen.

- ❖ Om Namo Bhagavate Vasudevaya
  - ➢ I bow in reverence to the Universal Guruh (God)
  - ➢ A calling to your Creator, not dissimilar to how a child calls the mother and the natural tendency for the mother to quickly tend to the needs of the child.

A Journey Toward the Unseen

If you have ever asked yourself, "Why am I here?" or "What is my purpose?", then at some level you are connecting with your inner self, your Soul. And if you have the ability to love yourself and others then you are connecting with Higher States of Consciousness, God or The Creator. If the highest goal for a human being is to become more conscious of these states, then how does one accelerate the rate of getting there?

Meditation (East) or contemplation (West) is our ability as an instrument of God to perceive through the realm of the seen into the realm of the Unseen, where the seen realm comprises our physical, mental, emotional, and ego states; and the Unseen realm comprises the Soul and God Consciousness. This ability occurs unconsciously in all humans as part of the evolutionary process to align their actions perfectly with the natural unfolding of the Will of God, so that love can be realized on Earth.

OPT2LIV.com is happy to share their doable three phase approach to Optimal Living, which has the potential to help one realize their pathway to the Unseen. To prepare for this journey it will be ideal for one to balance how they Breathe, Eat, Move, and Sleep.

If your goal is to move into Higher States of Consciousness one must first understand how to manage the physical. Let's break it down into smaller pieces: the evolution of the brain, the complexities of our mind, and our physical, and mental awareness.

Brain Development

The brain has evolved through three stages, 1) the Lizard Brain, 2) the Mammal Brain, and 3) the Human Brain. The lizard brain comprises the brain stem and cerebellum, which controls our fight or flight response, playing an important role in our survival as humans, but has little need in today's more civilized world. The mammal brain is composed of our limbic system, which controls our emotions, memories, and habits, and allows us to make decisions. The first two stages of our brain development are powerful aspects of our nature and where many of our obstacles arise. The part of the human brain that sets us apart from other animals is the neocortex. It controls language, abstract thought, imagination, consciousness, and allows us to reason. It is in this most recent stage of our brain development that we have the ability to realize our Creator consciously.

The Mind

Each person perceives the world around them through the mind. The following figure shows a simple depiction for how the mind perceives its existence, breaking it down into two distinctly different realms, physical awareness (seen) and Higher Consciousness (Unseen). The major components of our physical awareness include the physical, mental, and ego states. When these states are managed effectively there is a greater opportunity to connect with the Soul and God Consciousness. If not

195

managed, obstacles may arise that create substantial noise clouding our connection with the inner self.

In the following figure, notice that the physical awareness comprises more of the mind than our Higher Consciousness, this is because the amplitude of awareness is higher for the physical than that of the Soul or God Consciousness. As an example if the physical awareness was a rock concert then the Higher Consciousness would be a whisper. Therefore one will either need to figure out how to turn down the noise of the rock concert or master stilling the mind in order to attune oneself to the state of Higher Consciousness. But let's be honest, for most of us it will be easier to figure out how to turn down the noise, so let's focus on learning ways to soften, surrender and refine the physical awareness.

Physical Awareness
At the extreme of this noise exists chronic pain or the memory of a traumatic event. Both have the potential to create emotions that limit our ability to attune to the Unseen. Let's walk through what happens. The thoughts in the mind drive our emotions, which can trigger a primitive response that dumps chemicals in the body, turning on the sympathetic nervous system, and moving us even deeper into our physical awareness and further from the Unseen.

Please note that if you are currently suffering from a behavioral health condition that can not be self managed, please seek professional help. If you personally have the ability to safely self manage your mental state then it will be necessary to identify your triggers and use methods and practices to minimize their effects.

Mental Awareness

Our Mental Awareness comprises all of our memories, so finding stability here will depend on our ability to master concentration. This is the ability to focus our thoughts on one object for a prolonged period of time. This is a challenge for many today due to the endless distractions from media and technology. This is also where the memory of a traumatic event, if not properly managed, may present a lifetime of distractions.

Ego Awareness

As seen in the ego figure there is a mature ego and an immature ego. Typically we cycle through these states during our day but generally one or the other is our home base. The immature ego is divided into two sides, a low "i", which is someone that under identifies with themselves not realizing their identity and a high "i", is someone that over identifies with themselves like a narcissist. Both states have the potential to take us further from the Will of the Creator. Many times they initiate a primitive emotional response that fills the mind with dysfunctional desires to over control their environment or those nearby.

A meditation practice will help to form a mature ego, the true "I", giving an individual the opportunity to refine the working of the mind so that it operates at a higher vibration producing conscious thoughts that produce purposeful loving actions. We have seen many references of "dying to self to find self", meaning that the journey of consciousness begins after one releases their immature ego to find their mature ego. This removes the veil to the Soul and God, so that they may be clearly seen.

God Awareness
God is omnipresent, in us and around us at all times. To truly understand God Awareness our mind would need to understand the Infinite. Our brains today are mostly composed of our senses and a drive to survive. With the beginning of the evolution of the neocortex we are starting the process for realizing consciousness. If we are to truly realize God today we will need to go beyond the physical to experience the Unseen.

Thanks to quantum physics, science has now proven that there is more Unseen energy (96%, Planck principles) than seen energy (4%, Newton principles) in the universe. For many of us along a spiritual journey this Unseen and unmeasurable energy is God Consciousness, the Holy Spirit, Chi, or Prana to name a few, and is calling us to find our unique purpose in the universe, our Soul.

Soul Awareness
God, the collection of all things and energy in the universe and beyond, is infinitely organizing the unfolding of all of Creation. Our Soul is part of this unfolding and works to integrate with its human form, so that it consciously

realizes its purpose and/or how its actions today could perfectly align with the Will of God, not dissimilar to how a potter forms clay into a piece of art. If we walk this Earth consciously then we have the ability to perceive this connection, but many today are unconscious of this connection causing their actions to align with the lower energies of survival (fear, desire, and control).

Find and maintain a daily practice of meditation, so that your actions may perfectly align with the Will of God, creating a world full of peace, joy, and love.

Figure 1: Physical and God Conscious Images of the Mind

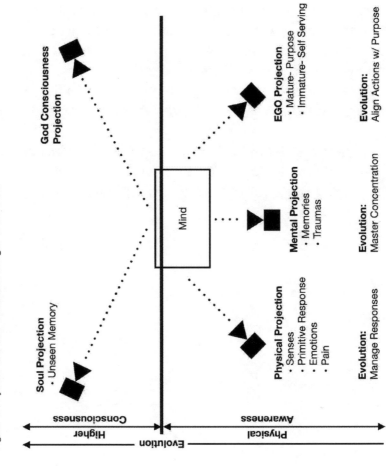

Figure 2: Physical and Soul Purpose Alignment

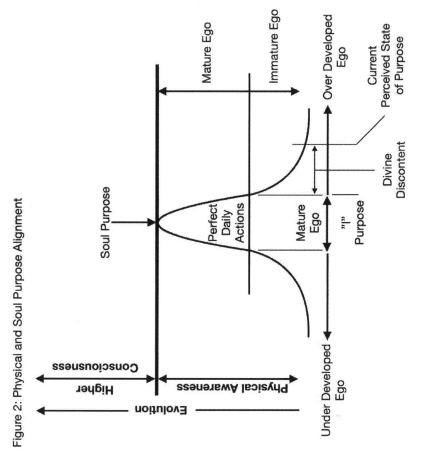